ENDLESS
energy

For Gail
with admiration and affection

A WORKBOOK FOR DYNAMIC HEALTH AND PERSONAL POWER

ENDLESS energy

For Women on the Move

SUSANNAH & LESLIE KENTON

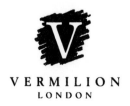

VERMILION
LONDON

Published in 1993 by Vermilion
an imprint of Ebury Press
Random House
20 Vauxhall Bridge Road
London SW1V 2SA

Third impression 1997

Catalogue record for this book is
available from the British Library.

ISBN 0 09 177753 4

Designed and typeset by
Write Image Ltd, London

Printed and bound in Great Britain by
Butler & Tanner Ltd, Frome and London

The material in this book is intended for informational purposes only. None of the suggestions or information is meant in any way to be prescriptive. Any attempt to treat physical illness should come under the direction of a competent physician who is familiar with nutritional therapy. Any serious psychological disturbance needs professional care. We are only reporters although we have had for many years a profound interest not only in how to look good and feel great as the years pass but in the fascinating and almost infinite capacity which women have to develop their creativity and experience joy. We write in the hope that some of our research may be of use to others who, like us, want to live long and well and to come into the fullness of their being.

Contents

Part one

The Process *of* Becoming

Health is a process of unfolding – the process of becoming who *you* really are. This journey towards endless energy asks that each of us discover her own path to wholeness.

Becoming a conscious traveller, a willing participant in your own journey can bring infinite gifts…

wellbeing…

personal beauty…

freedom…

Chapter 1

Energy *from* *the* source

Nothing gives a woman power so much as energy. It brings a light to your eye, a glow to your skin, an edge to your personality. When you are riding a wave of energy it seems to carry you wherever you want to go. When it crashes it can leave you feeling lost and lumpy. Energy is elusive stuff.

Working with women all over the world, hearing from them by letter, chatting with them over lunch, there is always one question that comes up: where do we get more energy? It is an important issue, a question we have wrestled with a lot in our own lives. It is also an issue which has particular relevance to women. Why? In the answer to this question lies the inner secret to accessing energy in its most powerful and fulfilling form. For as women, no matter how 'liberated' we think we have become, few of us live out fully who we really are. And it is only by doing *this* that you tap into the reserve of endless energy which lies at the very core of your being. This may seem a strange notion. After all, energy – the text books tell us – can only be measured in terms of calories. And what does *at the core* mean anyway?

When we say *at the core* we mean that part of you which is deeper than your personality. It encompasses your very essence. It is that in you which makes you unique from each and every person who ever lived and from which, when you know how, you can access universal life energy, directing it towards whatever ends you choose. More about all this later. As far as energy existing only as calories is concerned, any book or so-called authority who tries to convince you of this is either naive or sunk knee deep in the mire of nineteenth-century science.

Cycles of perfection

As a woman, the way you experience and express energy is more complex than a man simply because your biology is much more closely linked to nature's cycles – the waxing and waning of the moon, the movement of the tides, the energies of the earth, menstruation. To live at peace with yourself, to ride the waves of your biological, spiritual and emotional energy with grace and confidence (and to make the best use of all three), you need three things. First you need an awareness and a respect for the cyclic nature of energy and an appreciation for all of its different qualities. Secondly you need to know how to manage your energy when it needs managing – how to get down when you are strung up, how to heighten vitality when you feel low, and how to access stamina and sustained power for long-term efforts. Finally, and most important by far, you need to cultivate the art of living from your core – by dissolving any obstructions to the full expression of your beauty and authenticity. For there, at the deepest centre of your being, at the source of all your hopes and dreams, the fount of your own personal brand of endless energy is to be found. Tap into it and you begin to access a power for health, beauty, creativity and joy which is universal and yet which expresses itself in a highly individual way – as the uniqueness of you. This is what living with endless energy is all about.

Meet seedpower

Each woman, each human being, is utterly unique. Like the seed of a plant which has encoded within its genetic material the characteristics that will in time produce the full-grown flower, each of us comes into this world carrying a package of as yet unrealized but incredibly rich potential. We call this *seedpower*. This physical, psychic and spiritual potential creates each woman's uniqueness. She is rather like the individual brushstroke the zen painter uses to represent one leaf on a shaft of bamboo. The leaf he paints is totally singular – like no leaf which has ever existed. And yet within its uniqueness is encompassed universal beauty and life energy of the highest order. So it is with each human being. Within the individual genetic package which is you is nestled your very own brand of seedpower – a seedpower that encompasses far greater physical, creative and spiritual potential than any of us could hope to realize in only one lifetime.

Gardening good and bad

The remarkable thing about a seed is that very little is needed for it to develop into a plant: some good earth, rich in organic matter, some rain (not *too* much or the seed will rot), the sun (not *too* much or the young leaves will burn). These three simple things can provide the environment in which, thanks to its seedpower, the tiny plant grows into a full-blown flower.

People – you and us, and the man who works in the corner shop – are very much like plants. All we need is a good healthy environment which allows this unfolding to take place. The only problem is, more often than not the environment – physically, emotionally,

spiritually, socially – in which we grow does not support our full unfolding. And so, like a plant trying to develop in depleted soil with too little rain and too little sun, or a seedling trying to grow around a stone, we develop our own brand of *distortions*. These distortions can be physical – a sunken chest, poor posture, or an excess of fat created to cushion us against a harsh external world. They can be emotional – a sense that we cannot trust ourselves, intense shyness, lack of confidence, or a feeling of being unworthy or guilty. They can even be spiritual – a sense of meaninglessness which leads to addiction, a greed for material things which no matter how much you acquire never fills up the emptiness, a lust for power. Gradually such distortions become so much a part of our lives that we come to feel they are part of who we actually are.

Of course distortions are by no means all bad. Some help define our values. For instance a woman who has grown up in a family where she was continually treated as the scapegoat may develop a passion for helping the oppressed and make a fine career for herself as a social worker or political reformer. Someone raised on bad food who grew up constantly ill, like Leslie, may develop a fascination with finding out what kind of lifestyle promotes good health, and then spend much of her life helping to create it for herself and others. A woman growing up in a bourgeois family where social hypocrisy is the rule, in her rejection of it, may be driven to create a life for herself of breathtaking authenticity – perhaps as an artist who wrestles with the deepest human questions, in an attempt to bring her own truth into material form.

But there are also negative aspects to the distortions that develop when individual seedpower is thwarted. In some way each of us has been pushed too hard in an attempt to negotiate obstacles in our path. We've had too much responsibility, perhaps, inadequate nutrition, or hypercritical parents or teachers. Sometimes we have been born into a family with which, no matter how benign, we have little in common. As a result we can spend a lot of our lives feeling like a toad among ducks.

Energy thwarted

This situation – which tends to be the rule rather than the exception – can severely disrupt your ability to draw upon energy from your core. It also tends to produce artificial behaviour, like phoney personalities or false images, and psychic prisons into which we try to squeeze ourselves. A lot of energy which should be available for creativity, high-level health and joy, instead gets bound up trying to maintain these artificial creations. What is worse, this in turn can result in a sense of feeling separate from oneself, of not trusting yourself and of never being able fully to enter into what you are doing with joy.

In a woman it often creates a sense of not living comfortably in her own skin, feeling bad about her body and bad about herself, all of which makes her prey to eating disorders and to exploitation by our materialistic society. She is made to feel that being who she is, is not enough – that in order to be acceptable she has to change... to get thinner... drink a particular brand of coffee... wear certain perfumes... buy expensive clothes.

Woman rhythms

A woman's body is unique. Like a microcosm of the planet its rhythms ebb and flow in harmony with the changing cycles of time: the seasons, the earth and the moon, the hours of the day. The female endocrine system – which many scientists now believe to be the interface between spirit and body – is highly sensitive to external influences. Electromagnetic radiation in our environment – radio waves, nuclear fallout, even solar activity, as well as pesticide residues in our foods and heavy metals in the air we breathe – can all have a profound effect on our bodies and our psyches.

There is something magnificent in the way a woman in her wholeness resonates with the world around her. That is, when the environment in which she lives is *supportive*. The trouble is, our twentieth-century urban environment is often anything but supportive. Its plastic foods, its noise pollution, its emphasis on achievement without real concern for individual satisfaction, tend to create for the modern woman a world which drains her of her power. Then the energy rhythms through which she moves, instead of nurturing her, can antagonize her body in very real ways.

Here is but one of many scenarios possible: her immune system experiences environmental aggression alerting it to take defensive action. The white blood cell count rises, allergic reactions occur and red blood cells decrease, setting the stage for anaemia. From overwork or worry, a woman's body is flooded with cortisol and noradrenaline – stress hormones. In time this exhausts her adrenals and makes her body feel under constant siege. The result? Emotional upset, chronic anxiety or depression or physical exhaustion, premenstrual tension, early ageing, rheumatic conditions, or even more serious illnesses. Perhaps, too, she experiences hair loss, visual disturbances and rapidly ageing skin. For when a woman's energies are out of balance then her whole world is disrupted by the toxic condition of her body. And no amount of tranquillizers, champagne, love affairs or success in the outside world can compensate.

Journey to the centre

The process of rebalancing your body and reclaiming your energy means going to the core. It means rediscovering what you are all about beneath any distorted habit patterns you may have developed. (Here various techniques, some of which involve the active imagination, can be helpful.) It means reasserting your trust in yourself. It means, too, posing some interesting questions which can help make your own journey conscious. 'Who am I?' for instance and 'Where do I want to go?' It also means making use of simple but health-enhancing techniques – from new methods of exercise to nutritional and herbal supplements – all designed with one end in mind: to strengthen your core energy and enhance your body's metabolic processes.

For most of us such a journey demands that somewhere along the way we detoxify our bodies of the rubbish that may have accumulated over the years from poor eating, a sluggish lifestyle and a build up of internal toxicity from stress or living in a polluted environment. Even a simple spring-clean diet can help remove major blockages impeding the flow of core energy. Detoxification usually needs to take place on a psychological and spiritual level as well. Most of us carry around a burden of false ideas, notions and habit patterns – which either suppress or squander our core energy. They are false because they are not authentic to ourselves – they have not grown spontaneously out of our own seedpower. Instead they have been imposed upon us by our families, our religion, the cultural norms of our society. Such rubbish, in its own way, can be as big an energy-drainer as living on junk food. It too needs to be cleared away.

In this book we offer you some of the methods – both physical and mental – which we and the women we have worked with over the years have found useful in clearing away such rubbish, be it emotional, physical or spiritual. We also try to help you rediscover the unique nature of your personal seedpower using techniques for high-level health. They include special ways of exercising, eating and caring for yourself as well as new ways of looking at things and new approaches for relating to others. Everything in the pages that follow is here to help you develop the practice of *honouring* who you are. Do this and you can tap energy reserves which before now you may only have dreamed of.

Use it or lose it

The information, exercises, tools and techniques in this book are here for one purpose only – to serve *you*. *You* are not here to serve *them*. Frequently we meet women who say something like, 'I have come to your workshop because I have read all your books and I did what you said and I felt terrific… and then I got off the track … and I want you to get me back on track again.' Such women have a mistaken idea that they are somehow meant to be 'good little girls' doing everything the so-called experts tell them to get the rewards. Not only does such thinking rob a woman of her power, it belongs to the exploitive, energy-draining, freedom-limiting world which needs to be left behind if you want to draw upon endless energy from your own source.

Only *within* will you find the real expert on what is right and wrong for you, both in terms of high-level health and in how your individual nature needs to unfold. We hope that what we offer will help you clear away some of the static so you can more clearly hear the messages from your own inner expert when she speaks. What *works* for you will have done its job. Whatever doesn't work, please discard. Following anything slavishly never creates freedom. And individual freedom of the highest order is not only the key to lasting health, it is also a never-ending source of energy.

Workbook

for

Energy *from*

the source

Welcome to the workbook. There are two kinds of learning. The first is known as *conceptual*. It is the kind of learning that takes place in most schools. You hear about something, listen to and analyse the information, sift through what you think is or is not valid and then store away the facts in your brain where, hopefully, they may be of use to you later on. The second kind of learning is what is called *experiential* learning. Experiential learning can involve listening and taking in information too. But this aspect of it is not anywhere near as important as the testing of that information through experience.

Experience counts

Working with groups of people we often ask the question, 'What does trust mean to you?' There follows a discussion in which various participants put forward words to describe their ideas. One person may say, 'trust means being able to rely on someone, being safe.' Another says, 'trust is being sure,' or 'trust is letting go and knowing that it will be okay.' The opinions people offer are often interesting. They frequently deepen our own understanding of the word. But they are only *conceptual*. That is they are still part of the abstract world of thought. No matter how interesting or inspirational these concepts may be, they have very little power when it comes to transforming anybody's life. For conceptual learning remains in the head. All of us know people who are intelligent, and knowledgeable yet can never put into practice what they know to improve their own lives. Such are the limits of conceptual learning.

Knowing with power

Then we ask somebody from the group to stand up with their back to one of us. When they do, we request that they fall back into our arms promising that we will catch them. There follows worried laughter, hesitation and eventually letting it happen. Next we ask everyone in the group to stand up. Working with each other in pairs we get them to go through the same experience. Falling back into a partner's arms takes each participant way beyond conceptual ideas about trust into the realm of experiencing trust as a living reality.

One woman will stand up and throw herself boldly backwards, at the last moment panicking that nobody will be there to catch her. Another will hesitate, looking over her shoulder again and again, or will ask endless questions about whether it is possible to catch somebody who 'weighs as much as I do'. (In fact it is very easy even if someone is very big, provided you put your arms right under their shoulders. The more the person you are catching needs reassurance, the closer you stand to them.)

Each person's experience of this little exercise is unique and fascinating. If later you choose to analyse your own response it can tell you a lot about how you handle your life. But what is really important about all this is that every person who does it learns far more about trust from the exercise than they could learn in a month of Sundays sitting around talking about it. For they have *experienced* it. That is what *experiential* learning is all about. It is a learning which demands participation – personal involvement. Afterwards such learning becomes part of your being – body, mind and spirit. This alone removes it from the realm of abstract information and gives it power for transformation.

That is why we have chosen to create not only a book but also a workbook. We have designed it to bring you the experiential learning we find so exciting, even transformational, in workshops. It is our way of working with you as directly as possible. Experiential learning is the only kind that can lead you towards higher and higher levels of health, help you access your own brand of creativity and joy and put you in touch with your own source of energy.

How to use this book

Each chapter in this book is followed by a workbook or practical section which goes with it. It will contain questions, exercises, practical information and self-help techniques for you to explore. We would suggest you keep your own *Endless Energy* journal as you read through the book, and work through the questions and techniques to record your own insights, ideas and plans. This can be an A4 or A5 notebook you buy from any stationery shop.

Although it is possible to do some of the exercises mentally, the physical act of writing can be powerfully transformative. Both impatient readers ourselves, we know the tendency to skim through books and not bother with the practical parts. If this is your tendency too, we beg you in this case to make an exception.

In a workshop the process of personal transformation is enhanced and intensified by the interactions of the participants. Using a workbook, such transformation has to come from your personal interaction with the book itself. The results you get will depend to a great extent upon how much of yourself you are able to invest in this. Keeping a journal is the best way to maximize them.

Most of the exercises which require you to put pen to paper ask for no more than a few minutes of your time. Keep your journal close as you read so you can jot down your notes when an exercise comes up. You can go back to exercises which require more time when you have time to spare.

Bridge building

If you are one of those people who loves simple answers to simple questions, rather like multiple-choice exams, you may find working with your *Endless Energy* journal a very different experience. The value of keeping such a record lies not in giving the right answer to a question, but rather in the journal's ability week after week to expand your awareness, access your creativity and develop within you a feeling of what it is like to live more and more authentically. Such journal work has helped us and others to build important bridges between our inner world and the outer one in which we live and work, integrating the two and making us feel more whole.

Building such bridges takes time and patience. Each girder needs to be added one at a time. This can often mean learning to be still enough to hear your own messages from within. Many of us ignore such messages for so long that our inner voice becomes almost imperceptible. The exciting thing is that the more you act upon even the tiniest whispers from within, the stronger that voice becomes. In the process the bridges are strengthened so you can, with ever increasing ease, draw energy from the core and use it to create high-level health, personal beauty and the life you want.

Sometimes keeping such a journal means taking a good, hard look at things in your life you want to change and then committing to paper an intention to, say, make some alterations in your eating habits, make time to dance for fun, or explore the use of deep acting essential oils on your body. We suggest you record your commitments along with any insights that you have about yourself and your life as you fulfil them.

Your journal is *for your eyes only*. It is most definitely nobody else's business. So in creating it, give yourself total freedom. It doesn't matter what your spelling or grammar is like. It only matters that you take the time to write – logging your insights, your dreams, your intentions and your responses to some of the questions we will be asking in the book.

Quest for the core

The core of a human being can never be found by dissecting the human body. Nor can it be arrived at by analysing the human mind. But a sense of what we call living from the core is something each of us experiences at certain moments in our lives. In such moments we have a sense of simple bliss. Everything seems to fit together, or feel right, and life has meaning.

Some people express it as a sense of 'coming home'. Although most of us only happen upon this experience accidentally, it can also be cultivated by pursuing actions which make us feel good about ourselves and our lives. The techniques, information and exercises in this book are designed to help you do just that.

Sometimes, too, each of us inevitably loses touch with the sense of living from the core. Then life becomes extremely bleak and fragmented. Our only solace may be in remembering what it was like when we felt happy. At such times, making a leap of faith that everything will once again feel right is perhaps the hardest challenge any of us ever face. It is like the leap of faith which we are now asking you to take.

In the beginning even the idea that you have a core may seem farfetched. The notion that being connected with this core can bring a sense of meaning and happiness to your life may seem as fantastical as 'and they lived happily ever after'. But if you are prepared to take this first leap, the exercises in this book can help nurture this seed of possibility. Then, gradually, you can begin to experience your core as a powerful and highly personal reality – a foundation from which to live your own truth and draw upon endless energy.

Peak experiences

Use your journal to describe a moment or moments in your life where you felt the sense of living from your core described above. If you are not sure that you understand the idea of 'living from the core' simply describe a moment when you felt particularly happy. Remember the scene as vividly as possible and use as much detail as you can to recall your impressions. Use this description as a reference point from now on for how core connection feels for you.

Key questions

Ask yourself the questions below one by one. Then, letting your mind roam free, write down whatever comes to you. You may feel that one answer demands reams of words while another is very short. Be sure to explore each question fully before going on to the next. The questions are:

● **Who are you?** This does not mean your name and where you come from but rather what comes to your mind when the question is asked. How do you see yourself? What are you like?

● **What do you want?** This should include everything you feel you want or anything you secretly dream of, from the tiniest thing such as, 'I want to take up tapestry,' or 'I have always wanted to wear a red dress' to huge desires you may never have dared to voice: 'I want to go off to Africa to help native peoples dig wells' or 'I want to write a novel,' or 'I dream of being financially independent.' It doesn't matter, just write it down.

● **What do you *think* is stopping you?** Make a note of any circumstance, person, place, thing, thought or feeling that stands in your way.

We will be coming back to these questions and the answers you have recorded much later. But as you are going through the book you might from time to time want to look back at them and add to or change some of your answers. In our experience a person's answers frequently change as her awareness of herself and her values develops.

The process of going to the core is a very dynamic one which has its particular shape and its own direction. Your *Endless Energy* journal can be a powerful companion on the journey.

Chapter 2

Celebrating *the* body

How often do you rejoice in your body? How often do you feel at ease in your skin, at peace with yourself and in harmony with your world? For most women the answer is seldom. We tend to *put up with* our bodies as though they were slightly cumbersome things we have to carry about with us. Yet all thought, all feeling, every response to beauty and to horror comes through your body. It is your medium for experiencing everything in life. As any healthy two-year-old can show you, when *it* is fully alive *you* are fully alive. Such aliveness is central to an experience of endless energy. Young children have it naturally. Most of us have to rediscover it.

The body as object

Television, films and advertising are replete with photographs of long legged pencil-thin images which are supposed to be paragons of womanhood against whom we are asked to measure ourselves. Magazines and newspapers give a great deal of space to advice about diets, clothes and exercise supposedly designed to help our bodies more closely approach the shape, size and texture dictated as the fashionable ideal. Our crazy culture has created some pretty ridiculous and disempowering 'rules' for women – rules which act upon us often without our ever being aware of it.

American *Cosmopolitan* magazine once did an article informing readers how to have their sweat glands removed. They also offered advice on which sexual positions women can use to hide as many of their physical flaws as possible. They recommended the missionary position so long as the woman is underneath or propped up against a wall. They advised strongly against her being on top during sex lest her face droop and look unattractive. They also stressed the importance of keeping her arms at her sides so her breasts don't slip unattractively into her armpits. Meanwhile millions of women, because of their personalities, the way they are built and their own values (conscious or not), have not a hope in a million of ever 'getting it right' or looking like the 'ideal'. And they suffer.

This suffering goes deep – far beyond the simple yet painful feelings of inadequacy which come with having big feet or a flat chest, when the world tells you you are supposed to be different. Implicit in the whole way a woman's body is presented in our culture are two energy-draining assumptions: That the *body is separate from the spirit*; and that the body is *inferior*.

Anchored deep in our unconscious, these assumptions have evolved out of our Greco-Roman and Christian heritage which fears the irrational and the instinctual and glorifies the mind. They have created in us a nagging suspicion that our bodies are in some way not to be trusted – like a wild animal which must be tamed in size, in shape and in behaviour lest it get out of hand. This is particularly evident in the realm of eating and lies behind a growing incidence of anorexia nervosa and bulimia. Women suffering from either syndrome cannot even trust their own body to tell them when and what it needs for nourishment. So they become obsessed with consciously *controlling* appetite, terrified lest it run rampant through the refrigerator. The mind/body split is also responsible for a lot of unnecessary anxiety in women. And it has led us to look upon our bodies wrongly as physical objects – things separate from ourselves either to be prodded, criticized and hidden, or narcissistically exposed as sexual fodder.

The body as obsolete

Through all of this echoes a sense of woman's estrangement not only from her body but at a deeper level from herself. Out of this estrangement develops a sense of powerlessness which leads you to think that what you need to be happy, complete and fulfilled can only be found *outside* yourself – by accomplishment in the world, wearing the right clothes, earning a lot of money, winning the love of a man or conforming to some abstract ideal. Yet as long as you are driven by a sense of separateness from your body, whether you succeed or fail in getting what you think you want from the outside world is irrelevant. For neither success or failure brings you any closer to real satisfaction and fulfilment. Only wholeness can do that.

The energy of instinct

How does a woman reclaim her wholeness? By getting back in touch with the energy of instinct and giving it as much space in her life as she does reason. For any woman who lives by reason alone is only half alive. Rediscovering the aliveness of the child and the instinctual innocence of bodily freedom can not only help heal wounds of separation between instinct and intellect, it can go a long way towards freeing you to live in the fullness of your being. Being cut off from any part of yourself squanders energy – in anxiety, depression,

unfulfilling relationships, or fatigue or illness. Only when you come to live in wholeness do you have access to your full power. This means rediscovering without fear of self-indulgence how to celebrate your body.

Sex or sexuality?

Yesterday we bought a pile of women's magazines. They were jammed full of articles on sex. Each one talked not about the energy of instinct which fuels true sexuality but about the mechanics of the sex act: 'How To Make Oral Sex Work For You'… 'A Complete Guide to Sex Toys'… and so on. Like the perfect plastic models on the covers of glossy magazines, such information does little to help a woman reconnect with her body and reclaim the energy of instinct and her deep sexuality. It actually encourages her not to trust herself. It asks instead that she stand back from her body and judge it or that she put her trust in a lot of abstract how-to-do-it-better advice and commercial paraphernalia.

The ecstatic, irrational, primordial power of a woman can only be experienced and expressed in the kind of sexuality that enables her to forget the rules and let go of her rational mind, trusting for a time the impulses of her body. Instinctual energy is creation energy – the stuff out of which art is made as well as sexual ecstasy. So are joy and the sensual pleasures – taste and smell and sight and touch and sound. As we gradually connect with our instinctual selves and learn to trust them, a kind of alchemical marriage between instinct and intellect begins to take place and core energy from which we had been cut off becomes accessible. Such a marriage brings in its wake an experience of real personal power – the power with which each of us can create the life we want. When instinct and intellect are reunited, the body thrives. It helps protect against early ageing, increases vitality and heightens your capacity for joy.

There is only one problem. Like the wild fecundity of a rainforest (which is but another expression of the same life power), the instinctual energy of creation can be scary. It doesn't lend itself to rationalizations or structures. We will never understand it, neither can we comfortably put it into a little box to be dealt with when it is convenient. Yet instinct is a magnificent force. It needs to be honoured just as much as the power of reason. Each of us must find her own way to honour it, live it and express it. Otherwise it can turn in on itself and insidiously destroy the very fabric of our lives.

Reason and reptiles

Recent studies of the human brain have enabled scientists, probably for the first time, to chart biologically some of what takes place when we allow ourselves to surrender for a time to our instincts – in a sexual union, during an act of artistic creation, or in a state of deep meditation. Such experiences dissolve our sense of boundaries and allow us to merge into a celebration of simply *being* – of life itself. This can happen during childbirth. It can happen in what are sometimes called peak experiences as well. In all these cases we experience a sense of our own wholeness and of being connected up with the rest of life.

Each person in reality has not one brain but two. The rational brain or the *neocortex* is like an immensely complicated computer. It enables you to make conscious choices and to collect, store and interpret the data you receive from your sensory organs. The other brain, the subcortical nervous system or the *primitive* brain, is also sometimes called the *reptilian structures*. In evolutionary terms it is the oldest part. Unlike the conscious mind, it can never be dissociated from the basic adaptive systems on which survival depends.

Hormones and hardware

Your emotions and instincts are bonded to the activity of your primitive brain. Through the region known as the hypothalamus the primitive brain communicates by way of nerve cells with the rest of the body so that, thanks to complex feedback mechanisms, your hormones can regulate the activity of all the glands, organs and systems on which health and energy production depend. When you experience joy your hormonal balance is not the same as when you grieve or when you engage in intellectual thought.

In a truly healthy person the balance between these two brains is good. Unfortunately, however, the rational brain has the ability to inhibit the primitive brain. And in our modern world which elevates reason and denigrates the value of the body, this neocortical inhibition has been carried to extremes. As a result we have undermined our ability to experience ecstasy without drugs and have lost our trust in the knowingness of our instincts.

Take the experience of childbirth for instance. Instead of being able simply to give our body over to the event and trust that at the right time the appropriate hormones will be secreted to dilate the cervix and bring the child into the world, we try to exert conscious control over what is happening and to intervene in the process through reason. In doing so we inhibit the primitive adaptive responses on which birth depends and lose our trust in what is taking place. This causes hormones to shift in inappropriate ways. We lose touch with the ecstatic experience of surrendering the body to the birth process. We experience ourselves as separate from what is happening to our body and we feel pain. For we have brought into play the rational brain at an inappropriate time and we suffer for it.

It is not our highly developed rational brain that is at fault. Reason is valuable and necessary. It is the inappropriateness of allowing it to come into play at the wrong time which results in our sense of separation and anguish. For human instincts are fragile things – easily repressed, inhibited and changed by the power of the neocortex. In most of us the inhibition of instincts has become so unconscious, so habitual, that we are not even aware that it is taking place. We have simply forgotten how to let go and trust our body. Yet we have cut ourselves off from half of our being by suppressing the primitive brain. So instead of working with us, our instincts have come to work against us, depleting our life force and making us susceptible to depression, fatigue and dissatisfaction.

Being energy

To access endless energy – to live from the core – each woman needs a highly developed emotional and instinctive life as well as a good rational mind. We need to be able to trust the body and at appropriate times to abandon ourselves to it fully. Then the highly developed neocortex responsible for the development of culture and rational achievement ceases to work against us by inappropriate inhibition and serves instead to channel our instinctive emotional life in tremendously exciting and creative ways. We are able to experience joy in simply being, the way a child does. This is a joy and a radiance which does not depend upon what we do or what we have or on how clever or how admired we are – but simply on being.

Workbook *for* Celebrating *the* body

How does a woman re-learn to trust her body? How can she reclaim the power of instinct? Both involve listening, awareness and experiment. Both come slowly, in fits and starts, through real acceptance of your body as it is. When an instinctive impulse arises, *allow* it to happen. This is particularly important in the realm of sexuality where your primitive brain comes into its own more easily than in any other realm, provided you let it. Tapping into instinctual, creative energy demands that we re-learn to live *in* our bodies, respect what we *feel* with our flesh and behave with *kindness* towards it… hips and shoulders, breasts and legs and thighs – the lot. A growing awareness and acceptance of your body, regardless of size or shape, brings in its wake enormous personal power and the exhilarating experience of a freedom that is every woman's birthright.

Such freedom doesn't come in a ready-made pill you can pop. Neither can it be bought (despite advertisements which would have us believe it is as simple as owning a pair of Levi 501s or sipping white rum in a bikini on a white sandy beach). But there are a number of awareness games, simple exercises and instinctual 'indulgences' which have helped us a lot in our own search for greater freedom. Have a go with them. You might be surprised at how much they offer.

From your core

This little dance exercise is simple and fun. It is one of the best ways of reconnecting with your instinctual energies. For years, Leslie used it not only to connect with her body but also as a means of lifting away any emotional or physical stress that accumulated in her life. At times she danced for joy. At others she gently and finely let her body move. She sometimes danced in a frenzy of anguish or frustration, all the while simply allowing whatever was within her to pour through her body and out.

It is a technique we still use frequently when we are writing especially when words get blocked. We are always amazed at how affirming instinct through body movement releases energy you didn't even know you had.

Choose a tape or CD which you particularly like – one which touches your feelings. We often use primitive music from Africa or South America. After a while we find the rhythms in this kind of music take over so the body moves instinctively of its own accord.

Lock the doors and draw the blinds. Turn on the music. Stand for a minute or two in the middle of the room without your shoes and simply listen. Then slowly begin to *allow* your body to do what it wants. At first this may be very little. Be patient. Don't force anything. Soon you will feel some kind of movement arising from within. It might be nothing more than the flutter of one hand or a swaying to the beat. When it comes, follow it. For the next 10 to 30 minutes simply allow your body to move as it wishes – to dance, to sway, even to collapse on the floor if that is what it wants to do. Your job is only to give it the freedom to be itself instead of telling it what to do. If nothing happens after 10 minutes, don't worry. Next time, or the time after, it will. The point of this technique is not *what* happens but rather that you be *aware* of what is happening or not happening in your body.

Record in your journal what your experience of the exercise has been. What did you feel was happening in your pelvis? Your feet? Your belly? Your neck and breasts and face? The more you practice, the more easily your body will move. Few activities call forth instinctual energy like dance.

Reclaim your body

So many women dislike their bodies. When asked why, they say: 'I'm too fat' or 'I'm too thin' or 'my thighs are too big'. When asked, 'Compared to what?', they have difficulty answering. Some of the assumptions that women make about their bodies can be astounding. We recently overheard a tall, grasshopper of a woman we know compare herself with an athletic, amazon-like girl. 'Of course I am much heavier than she is,' she said. We looked at each other in amazement that her idea of herself could be so distorted.

Implicit in our culture is the idea of a right body shape. So insidious is this notion that we unconsciously and continually compare ourselves to a fictitious ideal. You don't have to continue to do this. Each woman has a choice. You can go on hopelessly *not* measuring up to a phantom, or you can get angry and quit. Only when you allow yourself to feel the injustice of trying to be what you think others want you to be, can you begin to reclaim the right to your own body. This exercise is designed to make you more aware of the attitudes to your body which you may be unconsciously carrying around with you.

Make a note in your journal of all the comments people have ever made to you about your body. Include criticisms you have made yourself. Let your mind range over the years but write it all down.

Here is an example of the kind of things one woman wrote:

Who does my body belong to???
When I was five my mother told me I couldn't wear a bikini because my tummy stuck out. She told me to hold it in.
My boyfriend tells me I'm too bony.
I think my bottom is too big.
I should be half a stone lighter.
My feet are ugly.

Now look at your list. How often do you notice the implicit presence of the notion of *right body shape*? How often in comparing yourself to this abstract idea do you come out the loser?

Body sculpting

Each of us does have our own right body shape – that is the shape encoded within our individual seedpower. Each of us also has distortions in that perfect form as a result of poor eating, negative self-image, neglect, lack of exercise and other factors. If not, you may be one of the lucky women who are pretty close to their own perfect form. To feel instinctively that the shape you are at this moment is not your 'true' shape is perfectly valid. Many of the exercise techniques and much of the advice about foods and eating in the chapters which follow are designed to help you uncover the true form hidden beneath the distortions.

To say 'I *hate* my thighs,' is something quite different. Ask yourself is it the thighs themselves or is it the distortion caused by the fatty deposits they carry that you dislike. Such thighs are nothing more than a sign that your body ecology is out of sync and needs attention. By using a spring clean diet, aerobic exercise, Power Toning (see p.113), skin brushing (see p.78) and a good anti-cellulite product, the thighs can change. But to *hate* your thighs is not only inappropriate, it can actually block you from being able to shed the stored wastes inside. Seeing distortions for what they are, stripped of their powerful emotional charges, empowers you to take the necessary steps to redefine your body's true form. But remember, the distortions which you so hate have developed out of an environment which did not offer your body the acceptance and support it needed – nutritionally, psychologically or in some other way. Real transformation – the kind of change that is permanent – only begins when you accept yourself for what you are and offer not criticism but loving care.

Carrying out the next two exercises – The Body Scan and the Revitalizing Breath – are good ways to begin. They can help you create a new relationship with your body, bringing awareness and new life to it and waking up areas that may have been 'asleep' for years.

The body scan

Every woman is more aware or feels more 'alive' in some areas than in others. This exercise can help you to find your 'dull' or 'dead' areas in order to consciously begin to integrate them and awaken your whole body.

You may want to record the following exercise on a tape recorder or ask a friend to read it aloud. Read slowly with plenty of long pauses between the words. It is important to take your time and feel what is happening.

● **Stand barefoot with feet shoulder width apart.** Notice the contact between the soles of your feet and the floor. Is your weight equally distributed or do you feel it more on your right foot or your left?

● **Begin with the left foot.** Ask yourself how much of your weight is on your heel? How much on the ball of your foot? How much is on the inner or outer edges?

● **Notice the arch of your foot.** Is it lifted or flat?

● **Now your toes.** Are they spread out or bunched up?

● **How does the very top of your foot feel?**

Now scan your right foot in the same way: notice the weight in the heel… the ball of the foot… the edges… feel the arch… the toes… the top of the foot.

● **Bring your awareness to your ankles.** Do they feel stiff or free?

● **Now travel up your calves to your knees.** Is there a difference between your right and left knee? Does one feel higher or tighter?

● **How do your thighs feel?** Is one more turned out than the other?

● **Notice the point at which your legs join your pelvis.** Is one hip higher than the other?

● **Become aware of the pelvis.**

● **Notice your buttocks.** Are they tight or relaxed?

● **Bring your attention to your perineum and to your genitals.** How do they feel?

● **Notice your belly. Be aware of the organs within it.** Are certain areas easier to sense than others?

● **Bring your awareness to your chest, your rib cage and your lungs.** Are you breathing more with one side or the other?

● **Look at your shoulders.** Is one more tense than the other? Is one higher or further forward?

● **Bring your attention to your back.** Beginning with the sacrum travel up to the middle back and then up to the neck. Do you notice any difference between the areas?

● **Now carry your awareness to your left arm.** Scan the upper arm and the elbow, the lower arm and the wrist. Sense your hand and your fingers.

● **Scan the right arm from the upper arm down to the finger tips.** Can you sense one arm more easily than the other?

● **Bring your awareness to your** neck. Sense the back of your neck and your throat. Is one easier to sense than the other?

● **Become aware of your head.** Notice your eyes and your eyebrows. Does one eye feel higher or more prominent than the other?

● **Sense your lips and cheeks.**

● **Notice your ears.** Does one feel more awake than the other?

Make a note of what you have discovered in doing the exercise. In particular write down any parts of your body which you had difficulty sensing. Did you notice a difference between your right and left side?

Different areas of the body often correspond to different aspects of ourselves. Compare your findings with the categories listed in Body Reflections in order to gain insight into the areas of your body or yourself that call for greater awareness or need strengthening.

BODY REFLECTIONS

Right side of the body. Corresponds to the more 'masculine' side of ourselves: rational linear thinking, assertiveness, authority, the father.

Left side of the body. Corresponds to the 'feminine' aspect of ourselves: emotional expression, instinct, creative thought, receptivity, nurturing, the mother.

Top half of the body. Corresponds to our expressive, outgoing, social, active aspect.

Bottom half of the body. Corresponds to our more private, introspective, home-loving, supporting, stabilizing aspect.

Front of the body. Corresponds to our conscious self and the social persona.

Back of the body. Corresponds to our unconscious self and the inner being.

Sometimes when an area of your body has suffered trauma through an accident, or rape, or an operation it can be very difficult to bring your awareness into it. A woman who has had an abortion, for instance, may feel that her entire pelvic region is dull or cut off. Once you identify such an area with the scanning exercise you can then re-invite awareness to it using the Revitalizing Breath.

For instance, if you found it difficult to sense your left side, or if you often suffer pain in the left side of your body, it may be that your rational or 'male' side is overly developed. You may have learnt to be very much in control and assertive and as a consequence your 'female' side may have been neglected. If this is the case, you could look for ways of allowing your creativity greater expression.

Revitalizing breath

This technique makes use of the power of the breath to bring awareness and life back to 'cut off' or neglected parts of your body. By focusing your breath consciously in a neglected area you can bring energy to it. As you do this over a period of time you gradually enable the area to become re-integrated with the rest of your body. And each step you take towards integrating a neglected part of yourself brings you access to more core energy.

Imagine your breath as the gift of life. As it flows into your body it brings you fresh life energy. As it flows out it removes anything stale or old – such as physical waste or unwanted thoughts and feelings.

Make yourself comfortable lying down and become conscious of your breathing. Don't do anything to change it, simply listen to it for several breath cycles. Then, after an exhalation pause, prepare a warm space in your body to welcome the life-giving breath. Receive the breath into the space and feel it filling you with its energy. Imagine that as it flows out again it removes any wastes with it. Once you understand the principle of the Revitalizing Breath you can invite it into any area that feels dull or damaged. Simply focus your awareness in that place, then create the space to welcome and allow each inhalation and exhalation. You may want to lay your hands on the area to help guide the breath where you need it.

Make a note of your impressions in your journal. Was it easy to *allow* the breath or did you find yourself *trying* to breathe? Can you describe in your own images the sensation of the breath flowing into and out of your body? Did this exercise conjure up any feelings for you?

Body nurturing

Many of us only notice our body when it causes us pain or discomfort. We blame it when it lets us down through injury or sickness. We chastise it for not being the right shape or size. At best we ignore it. But how often do we approach our body with a sense of gratitude for supporting and protecting us? For translating our desires into actions? For allowing us to experience a myriad of feelings and sensations which bring meaning to our life? Here is the chance to make amends. Show your appreciation for your body and nurture it with experiences that bring it bliss.

List in your journal all the things that bring pleasure to your body. Then commit yourself to enjoying one or more of these things within the next 24 hours. When you indulge in the experience – really go for it. See just how much enjoyment your body can take! Here are a few of our favourites:
- Eating fresh lychees and mangoes
- Making love
- Running along the cliffs above the sea
- Lying on one's back in the middle of a sunny field
- Smelling lilies and freesias
- Giving and receiving good hugs
- Body surfing in the waves
- Being massaged
- Feeling the breeze on one's face on a motorbike ride
- Swimming naked
- Nursing a child
- Lounging in front of an open fire
- Listening to the purr of a cat

Blissful self-massage

The next time you get out of the bath or shower, treat yourself to 5 minutes of massage with a delicious body oil or lotion. As you apply the oil, be aware of each part of your body in turn. Notice how it feels beneath your hands and how your hands feel to your body. As you touch each part of you, approach it as you might when looking at the fine veins in a flower petal, in admiration for the magnificence of nature.

Working with any of these exercises over the next few days and weeks you will find that your body begins to 'speak' to you about what it wants and needs. Listen to and honour it. Record in your journal some of the 'messages' it gives. You may be surprised at how much it has to say – surprised, too, at the way in which this listening and honouring of your body helps bridge the gap between instinct and intellect. It can also bring you a wonderful new sense of personal power and self-confidence, not to mention connecting you up with deeper levels of energy with each week that passes.

Chapter 3

Free *your*

spirit

J ust as you need to reclaim your body for full access to core energy, you also need to make full use of the remarkable powers of your mind. For it, more than anything else, can help free your spirit. Mind and body, far from being two separate entities are really opposite ends of the *bodymind* continuum – two aspects of the same living being which is you. This notion of bodymind as a single entity may seem strange to you. For we have grown up in a culture that has long ignored mental and spiritual influences in its attempt to reduce the phenomenon of life to mere random chemical and physical events.

The materialist worldview

A worldview is a way of looking at the world which remains unconscious in a culture but which tends to govern the judgements we all make as part of that culture. It is a kind of unspoken consensus about reality. Whether or not you are a scientist, whether or not you have read the philosophers out of which our materialist worldview has evolved, it nonetheless affects you. It is etched deep into the fabric of the unconscious assumptions that govern how we live our lives.

Until the seventeenth century an experience of the unity of mind and body formed an integral part of people's belief systems and healing practices. An awareness of bodymind existed as far back as ancient Egypt and before. Ayurvedic medicine (the oldest known system of healing in the world) is based on it. So are Chinese medicine and spiritual healing. Then in eighteenth-century Europe, after the onset of the Industrial Revolution and following in the wake of Descartes and Newton, our worldview changed. We began to view men and women as a blend of mechanism and egotism. We started to see all phenomena in the universe, even life itself, as nothing more than a collection of complex, yet ultimately explainable, random chemical and physical events, and we insisted that the whole is nothing more than the sum of its parts. We also came to look upon ourselves as quite separate from the world around us, rather arrogantly assuming we would be able to make indiscriminate use of the earth's resources to further our own purposes. It is an assumption which, in the face of the ecological crisis threatening our planet, we now know was a highly dangerous one.

In lots of ways our mechanistic worldview has been useful, especially for science and technology. It has enabled us to study and organize experience – to categorize different species of animals and to develop steam engines.

The only problem is that, as we now know, it has serious drawbacks. It does not take into account enough of reality. It teaches us to look at life as something built out of minute particles. This in turn leads to an assumption that, provided we know enough about these particles, we can take them all apart and then put them all back together to make life. Sounds great. Except it doesn't work. Take an apple for instance. You can analyse and measure its chemical content, its vitamins, minerals, natural sugars, fibre and so forth to the nth degree. Yet no matter how hard you try to mix these ingredients together again you can never make an apple. Only life can do that.

Personal and planetary disasters

Our limited worldview has led us to exploit the resources of our planet without regard for the consequences of our actions – bringing about the thinning of the ozone layer as a result of CFC release and destroying our rainforests. In the areas of personal health it has also wreaked havoc with our lives. For twentieth-century medicine, instead of honouring bodymind and taking into account the effect of our mental and spiritual life upon the immune system and our ability to resist degeneration, has opted for a naive symptomatic approach to treating illnesses. Using powerful drugs designed to alleviate one condition can cause serious side effects and create other illnesses. It can also unbalance body energy and contribute to degeneration. Western medicine has not recognized that thought and substance, like mind and body, are only different aspects of the same universal energy. It was only physicists and mystics that understood this.

The big crunch

Einstein observed that matter and energy are interchangeable. Quantum physicists went further. They showed that the 'particles' out of which we believed the universe to be built were not as solid as we thought. Experimenting with atoms, they discovered that sometimes electrons appear as particles and at other times as waves. Then came the crunch which shattered the mechanistic worldview into a million pieces: these same scientists were stunned to find that whether an electron appeared as a particle or a wave depends

entirely on how they *expected* it to appear. They discovered that the power to alter reality amazingly comes from the *mind* of the observer.

This discovery forced physicists and biologists to revamp their vision of reality and to acknowledge the interconnectedness of all things and the power of consciousness to change reality. Now, inexorably, almost a century later, it has begun to transform health care. Once health and illness were seen as separate entities visited upon us through the powers of fate which only medical intervention could help. Now they are increasingly viewed as intricately related to our lifestyle, feelings and state of mind, as well as (like the shape-shifting electron itself) to what consciously or unconsciously we expect to happen to us.

Bodymind connections

For generations there have been those who preached the power of mind to influence body. Only recently have researchers begun to draw scientific maps of *how* this happens. Most of the new knowledge comes out of a fascinating medical and biochemical discipline with an absurdly long name: psychoneuroimmunology – or PNI for short.

PNI is the scientific study of bodymind. Leading researchers in the PNI field, such as Dr G.F. Solomon at the University of California, have discovered that the human mind (which includes our conscious thoughts and unconscious impulses as well as our super-conscious or transcendent mind and our emotions) is elaborately interwoven with every function of the body via nerve pathways and chemical messengers – the endorphins, neuropeptides and hormones. A hormonal-nerve relationship exists between your endocrine glands, via the pituitary (master gland regulating the actions of all others), the adrenals (which deal with stress) and the hypothalamus. It is called the hypothalamic-pituitary-adrenal-axis and it links your thoughts and emotions with physical responses. New evidence even suggests that, rather like the physicists' electrons which appear as either waves or particles depending upon expectations, your body's chemical messengers – the neuropeptides – may be made up of a single molecule whose configuration can be altered by your mental, emotional and spiritual state, to create new forms. With each passing month more scientific maps of bodymind are being drawn. They show how what you think and feel powerfully influences the levels of vitality you experience, as well as how slowly or rapidly you age, and whether or not you are able to resist infections.

Mindbending

In a laboratory at the School of Engineering and Applied Science at Princeton University in the United States sits an interesting electronic device known as a *random-event generator*. It issues positive and negative impulses in a random way. It is really nothing more than a machine for tossing coins electronically. According to the old worldview there is no way in which your mind can influence an electronic machine to behave in any way other than the random way in which it has been programmed. Yet lengthy experiments with a great many people have shown just the opposite. They indicate that when you focus your mind for a certain length of time on influencing the random-event generator to produce more positive signals than negative ones (or vice versa) that is just what happens to a *statistically significant* degree. This is but one of many such leading-edge experiments which indicate that how you think affects not only your health and the quality of your life but also *external* reality.

Through our consciousness we appear to be linked via complex energetic interfaces with other living organisms and non-living things – even the planet itself. Becoming aware of these interfaces – connections which are now being mapped by brain researchers, psychologists, spiritual leaders and high level physicists – can open up a whole new sense of personal freedom. It can make you aware that as a human being you are *not* trapped inside some mechanical universe from which you can never escape and over which you exercise no personal choice. You have, through your own consciousness, a power that can help change the universe and recreate your own life. The important issue then becomes: how do you put that power to work to help free your spirit?

Quantum mind

Transpersonal psychology and the humanistic inner-disciplines hold clues. They work with the modern mind in ways which often coincide with ancient wisdom from the world's great spiritual traditions. When we say 'mind' by the way, we mean not only your conscious everyday mind that remembers to empty the rubbish and call a friend, but also your subconscious. The subconscious mind is full of feelings, memories, dreams and dramas. It also encompasses the *knowing* necessary to run your body, make sure you breathe when you need to, break down wastes and eliminate them and build new hormones and cells and tissues – all of which happen without your having to pay the slightest conscious attention to what is going on.

The unconscious mind can be tremendously useful when it comes to helping release core energy for use in your life. The trouble is, the unconscious frequently gets clogged up with a lot of negative beliefs, fears and self-limiting shadows from our past. These things need to be made conscious or they can greatly impede energy-flow from the core. We will be looking at how you can help your unconscious detoxify these energy-drainers and blockers later on in the book.

To tap into endless energy from your core (not to mention to prevent the kind of environmental destruction which could well eliminate the human race) we need to expand our vision of reality. We need to develop a new, broader, and more appropriate worldview – one which helps free the spirit. Such vision takes time to evolve of course, but gradually it becomes incorporated into our unconscious. Then, instead of *limiting* our ability to care for ourselves in optimum ways, it can empower us to do so.

Worldview for freedom

The new worldview needs to encompass some very important ideas which only a few years ago would have seemed absurdities to the average person: an awareness of the interconnectedness of mind and body between ourselves and others, and between us and our planet. This new way of looking at life includes a growing sense that somewhere deep within us is a *knowing* beyond the limits of conscious awareness. Provided we are willing to experiment with that knowing and willing to look beneath the surface we can, each of us, discover new solutions to old problems, free blocked creativity and achieve levels of physical and emotional wellbeing that would otherwise be far beyond our reach in the stress-filled and polluted environment in which we live. What the two of us find especially exciting about all this is that this expanding awareness developing out of modern science and philosophy increasingly empowers us as individuals and helps us learn how to live from the core. It also helps us become more effective in making our individual contributions to life outside of us.

You have a great friend in your unconscious mind. Once you start to respect it and learn how it works, you start to draw on its almost infinite power for healing, transformation, problem-solving and (best of all) creativity. By creativity we not only mean being able to write or paint, or arrange flowers or play music, but being able to make your dreams a reality.

Learning new skills

The unconscious works in a very different way to its conscious counterpart. Your conscious mind is critical, focused and rational. It can only deal with one thing at a time. Your unconscious knows no such barriers. Psychologists and other researchers who have examined how unconscious processes behave have discovered that the unconscious has no space/time limits. It does not separate what it experiences as happening now with what it experienced from earlier times nor even from what may come into being in the future.

The unconscious also does not differentiate between a real event and an imagined one. It is this characteristic which is such a nuisance when we are experiencing our own negative shadows from the past. You know the kind of thing: say, when you were a child you once fell off a high bed hurting your head badly. The head is long healed but the *feeling* from the experience still rests somewhere in your unconscious so that every time you go into a bedroom where there is a high bed you feel uneasy.

That is the down side. This timelessness and inability to differentiate between what is imaginary and what is real has an up side, too, which makes it especially useful in helping you release core energy. Unlike the conscious mind which measures every thought with which you present it against external reality, the unconscious measures what it is offered only by the intensity of the image or experience it evokes. How vivid is it? How much emotive power does it carry? These are the criteria your unconscious uses in deciding to move into action or not. And when it plays upon an intense image often it can bring what it is imagining into being.

In recent years the capacity of the unconscious to bring about whatever you give it to imagine has been much used by sports coaches. To improve performance they get their athletes to sit or lie down, shut their eyes and daydream, imagining themselves, say, clearing the high-jump set higher than ever before. It has also been used with biofeedback training in teaching people to evoke the help of their unconscious mind to alter blood pressure that is too high or dissipate an agonizing migraine by imagining their hands growing warm, thus drawing congested blood out of the head and ameliorating the pain. The key to making use of this superb imaginative power for yourself is twofold.

First you have to provide your unconscious with vibrant images of what you want to create – images it loves to play on whether they be words, or visual pictures, or even vague longings. Whatever they are these need to be images you find exciting, pleasing, fun. Second you must allow your mind to play with these images *often* while in a deeply relaxed state *again and again*.

This way, using repetition and evocative words, images and thoughts, your unconscious mind's ability to alter your life for the better appears almost unlimited. The unconscious can enable us, if we so choose, to clear out limiting false beliefs and ancient emotional shadows that stifle. It can help us change whatever we want to change, heal whatever we want to heal and even create things which for years we have been longing to create against all hope. Not to work with the simple yet powerful techniques which spur your unconscious into action is like trying to live your life with one hand tied behind you. Learn to work with its energy in simple ways. (Remember the power of experiential learning for transformation?) Then use these techniques in an exercise or two each day. It will not only help free your spirit. It can make it soar.

Workbook

for

Free *your*

spirit

Having the experience of bodymind so it becomes a living reality for you, instead of only an abstract concept, is an important step in freeing your spirit. For part of the split between mind and body is the common experience of not feeling all in one piece – unable to rise spontaneously to whatever challenge you have chosen for yourself. Here, some exercises for neurosensory integration can be useful.

Another way to bring about bodymind integration is to learn a technique which activates the powers of your conscious mind, and then practise it together with another designed to trigger unconscious strengths, both of which you will find in the Tune in – Turn On section which follows. When you direct these exercises towards the end of honouring your own integrity and releasing core energy you create a power-house of mind energy in the service of your own positive transformation.

Finally, we like to use a technique which we call writing from the core. We find it can help you to get in touch with and *externalize* your spirit and sharpen your senses so that you experience the world around you with the freshness of a child. Let's look at sensory integration first.

Brain games

Neurosensory integration (NSI) is scientific jargon for the wonderful feeling you have when you know you have *got it all together* – when your brain, nervous system and body are working well and everything seems right.

Neuro-hardware

Your brain not only has many different parts – from the highly evolved neo-cortex, seat of abstract thought, to the limbic system by which we are linked to our reptilian ancestors through our instincts – it is also divided into two hemispheres, left and right. These hemispheres are separated by the corpus callosum, a membrane which, being electrosensitive, translates incoming nerve messages and re-directs them for action in the body. The corpus callosum is the area of the brain that can (and often does) get overwhelmed from eating, or too much stress, emotional pressure, electromagnetic or chemical pollution, negative beliefs about yourself, or even fatigue after pushing yourself too hard for too long. These things cause chemical residues to build up so that this important membrane loses sensitivity and can result in poor coordination in your body, or a sense that harmony is missing from your life. Then you are less able to experience deep connection with your world through touch, smell, taste, hearing and sight.

Games for neurosensory integration are physical techniques that help link all parts of your brain (with its intellectual, instinctual and imaginative functions) to your body and to the world around you via your senses. Practise them regularly to get to know them, then use them whenever you particularly need help in gathering yourself. They can enable you to come to experience your own bodymind and know how it operates as a single entity.

Many of the NSI games are so effective because they help

re-establish energetic balance in the corpus callosum, bringing about good connections between the brain's two main divisions: right and left. These divisions are by no means cut and dried. Research indicates, however, that your left brain tends primarily to deal with rational processes of linear thinking. Your right brain tends to experience reality more intuitively, to be more involved with creative energies, and to establish patterns of interrelatedness between things, feelings and ideas.

In the West we are trained through the values implicit in our educational system to be left-brain thinkers. Overvaluing the rational and focusing too much on left-brain skills tend to cut us off from our instincts and to limit our capacity for joy, energy and creativity. It can lead us to an existential sense of meaninglessness as though we are leading deadened lives, not fully satisfied with work and relationships nor able to involve ourselves fully in the world around us.

Mind integration

The simple techniques below rely on physical movements to re-establish a free flow of energy between right and left hemispheres via the finely tuned corpus callosum. Try them for 5 or 10 minutes a day. Record any feelings or experiences they bring you in your journal. Once you get the hang of doing them, they become like old friends whom you can go to for help when you need it. All of them regulate electrical interfaces in your nervous system gradually helping to re-establish a sense of balance and harmony.

Left or right dominant

Before you begin, try this exercise to find out which part of your brain tends to be dominant.

Using a sharp pencil, make a hole in the centre of a blank piece of paper. Hold the paper at arm's length and look at an object on the other side of the room through the hole. Focusing on the object, slowly bring the paper towards your face. You will naturally bring the hole towards your dominant eye. Now close first one eye and then the other. The eye with which you can still see the object through the hole is the dominant one.

The next two exercises are super tools for linking up right and left hemispheres and establishing balance between them. Practising them regularly helps integrate intuitional and intellectual thinking with body movement and sensory experience. They also help bring a sense of harmony and ease to whatever you do.

Cross links

This exercise consists of three sets of movements to be repeated a dozen or more times at your own pace. (We sometimes do them to music or while bouncing on a rebounder.)

Bend your right arm and lift your left knee, touching the elbow to the knee. Do the same thing on the opposite side touching your left elbow to your right knee. Repeat 4 times.

Now similarly touch your right hand to the bottom of your left foot. Then bending your right leg, touch your right foot with your left hand. Repeat 4 times.

Bend your left leg and swing it behind you to touch your right hand to your left sole. Then swing your right leg up behind you to touch your left hand to your right sole. Repeat 4 times.

These 3 exercises make a set. Repeat each set as many times as you need to to feel the effect. You can do the exercises slowly and gently or in a very lively way almost leaping up and down. Discover which rhythm suits you best each time you do them. (We *love* to laugh while doing it too!)

Cross sit-ups

Lie down on your back and bend your knees. With your hands behind your head bring your right elbow to your left knee and then your left elbow to your right knee. (This is also good for toning tummy muscles.) Touch each elbow to the opposite knee twelve or more times.

Tracing infinity

This simple exercise stimulates the cerebral cortex while helping to integrate right and left brain functions as well. It is a gem when you are getting ready to perform any creative task or intellectual process such as writing a report. Its simplicity belies its power to get your mind and body humming in harmony and all directed towards the same end.

Put the palms of your hands together and clasp your fingers. Straighten your two index fingers to make a point. Standing with your feet comfortably apart, use your pointed fingers to trace a large infinity sign (or a figure eight) in the air in front of you. As you trace, follow the movement with your eyes. Make sure that the direction you trace in is always up through the centre of the figure. Do the exercise for a minute or two.

Lazy lunges

This little technique is ideal for helping to focus your bodymind on whatever you happen to be doing. It is also a wonderful way of grounding yourself after any emotional upset or in the midst of confusion.

Spread your legs comfortably, pointing your right foot straight ahead and your left foot to the left at a 90 degree angle. Breathe out while bending your left knee. Then breath in as you straighten your left leg all the while keeping your back straight. Repeat this three times then change legs and repeat.

Tune in – turn on

Here are 2 simple exercises far more powerful than all the leading edge information about exercise and nutrition when it comes to releasing energy and integrating all the different parts of your being. The first one activates your conscious mind using the rational words it understands. It is done a few times during the day whenever you think of it. The second one develops the powers of your unconscious mind. It is only done when you are in a state of deep relaxation.

Make conscious choices

These are choices you make consciously with full awareness. It is perfectly normal to have doubts while you are repeating these choices to yourself. This has no bearing at all on their usefulness in helping you to tap core energy. Make the following 4 choices – repeating each 3 times silently to yourself several times a day whatever else you may be doing:

> *I choose to be whole*
> *I choose to be free*
> *I choose to be true to myself*
> *I choose to trust life*

Play with images

Allow your imagination to play with these words silently in a state of deep relaxation. You can do this just before sleep, if you awaken in the middle of the night, on waking up first thing in the morning for 2 or 3 minutes, or any other time of the day or night when you can close your eyes for a few moments and let your imagination flow with whatever images the words bring up. The more you play with them and enjoy them, the more quickly and dynamically will your unconscious mind be spurred into creating them as part of the living reality of your world.

> *I am whole*
> *I am free*
> *I am true to myself*
> *I trust life*

That is all there is to it. You might like to record in your journal any particularly clear or pleasing images that come out of this exercise. You may also want to record any thoughts or feelings (positive or negative) which the practising of either brings up. Just write them down and leave them. We cannot describe to you how integrating and transformative these 2 exercises are. You need only continue to repeat them each day to experience their effect.

In the beginning, when you are not used to connecting with your unconscious mind in this way, you may find doing so seems to drag up a lot of cynical thoughts or negative feelings like sadness or resentment. This is a normal part of linking in to your unconscious. It is as if by doing this you give it the right to clear out all the old rubbish it has been carrying around. Don't worry about it if this happens to you – just let it come to the surface, make a note of it and get on with the exercise as you go about your daily life. Be a little patient. It takes a bit of time to mobilize your unconscious if until now you have looked upon it not as a friend but some kind of scary underworld which you have tried your best to stay out of.

Writing from the core

The greatest challenge to living from your core is discovering the uniqueness of your own being. At the beginning of the workbook you answered the question 'Who are you?' Take a look at your answers. Do they indicate that your sense of self comes from the way you dress? How you look in the mirror? The job you do? The roles you play as a mother, a wife, a girlfriend, a sister, a daughter?

While it is true that any of these things *can* help define us, they only give a partial and often transitory sense of self. For instance, a woman who defines herself as a mother, when her children grow up and leave may feel completely lost. Or a dynamic working woman who loses her job may feel as though she doesn't exist without it. Any sense of your self which relies entirely upon the external circumstances of your life can pass away. Be prepared.

You are unique

Finding a vehicle for self-expression such as writing can help you build the foundations for a whole new sense of self. This is because writing, like painting, sculpting and other creative activities, helps you to get to know yourself from the inside out. Then, instead of relying upon the mirror, your relationships with other people or your job to give you a clue as to what you are like, you begin to see and experience yourself firsthand. The act of creative writing also keeps you in touch with your inner world and develops your own *voice*. As you express this voice on the page, you make visible your individuality.

In the beginning you may find your inner voice shy and difficult to coax out. You may also be disappointed when you read the words you have written. But, gradually, as you lose yourself in the fun of the writing process you will find that the inner voice emerges of its own accord with increasing boldness and confidence. Then, after a month or so you may be surprised to look back on something you have written and say, 'Did I really write that? It's good!'

Just as in the section Tune In – Turn On, when you trained your conscious and unconscious to work together to help brain and body to become more integrated, so the act of writing regularly helps build a bridge between your inner and outer worlds. The more these worlds connect, the more authen-

ticity you have and the more living from your core becomes secondnature.

As we said in Chapter 1, Energy From the Source, keeping a journal of your thoughts, feelings and discoveries is the best way to get the most out of the *Endless Energy* journey. We have found writing to be such a powerful tool for self-transformation, that we encourage women to make a daily practice of it. Such a practice is an important way of allocating 'self time' devoted to your own unfolding. Many busy women, in fulfilling their various roles as working woman, mother and wife, forget to take time out for themselves. Yet setting aside just 15-30 minutes a day to write can help you access hidden reserves of personal energy and burn off excess stress.

Banish writer's block

Before you even begin to write, the fear of the blank page can block you. Writer's block is something we both find very amusing. Not that we haven't at times suffered real anguish from it ourselves, but ever since we met Eva we have never been able to complain of writer's block without smiling at the absurdity of it all.

Eva came from California. She lived with her wealthy husband in a beautiful house overlooking San Francisco Bay in Marin County. When we were introduced as writers, Eva told us that she too was a writer. We asked what she wrote and Eva told us that in fact she hadn't written anything for the past four years. At first she said, this had concerned her, but now everything was okay. She had found a terrific writers' therapy

group and, after a year of attending it, she told us enthusiastically, she knew the *reason* she had produced nothing. She was, she informed us with a completely straight face, suffering from 'writer's block'.

Anyone who sits down to write for the first time experiences some form of writer's block. This is because our capacity to judge and criticize is so much more strongly developed than our ability to allow ourselves to just *be* and have fun. Before we have even written the first letter we are already wondering – will this be any good? The best bet is to assume that it won't be. But who cares? Here for once in your life is a place where anything you do is all right. The process of expressing yourself matters much more than the words you produce. Affirm your right to put down whatever you want and to make lots of mistakes. When you learn to make them, with impunity, you will be on the right track.

To get a taste for what writing from the core has to offer, promise yourself to sit down and write for 15-30 minutes every day for a week. Make a decision not to *read* what you have written during that week nor to *judge* yourself as you write. Accept that as a novice you have *carte blanche* to put down absolutely anything.

Find or buy a pen and notebook that you enjoy writing with. You may like to write in purple ink, with a fountain pen, a felt tip, or a propelling pencil. Maybe you prefer lined paper, maybe plain, a ring-bound notebook or a loose-leaf binder.

Give yourself the freedom to write whenever and wherever you please. Be imaginative in your choice of place. Try your kitchen, a park bench, a tea room, a hotel lobby, a train, the bath, a restaurant while waiting for someone. Find time during your lunch hour or on the way to a meeting, first thing in the morning, or last thing at night. Let the time and place inspire you

What to write

Deciding what to write can seem a stumbling block. It needn't be. Remember, anything goes. Write about your favourite place or person, a wonderful night out, your most embarrassing moment, an act of kindness that touched your heart, how you felt (or feel) at the betrayal of a lover, the secret life of your greengrocer, a scene you witnessed on the way to work, how your body feels right now, an incident that made you really angry, a conversation you over-heard in a restaurant, learning to write at school. If none of these interest you, play the word game: pick subjects at random from your imagination – alligator, salami, camping, turquoise sequins, full moon. Then select a word and spin out any thought, feeling or memory connected with it. Amuse yourself! As each day that you write passes you will find that topics automatically suggest themselves or even *demand* to be written. You may be walking somewhere when you suddenly have an idea for a short story or you may meet a person that you want to write about. When you think of a writing topic, make a note of it and store it in a list at the back of your notebook to draw upon later.

Decide how long you will write each day, put your pen to paper and go. Don't stop until your time is up. The less you pause the more free, spontaneous and enjoyable your writing will be. Do not read back over what you have written, don't cross anything out and don't give a second thought to your spelling or handwriting.

Most of us have a strong Inner Critic who is ready to pounce on any attempt at self-expression and sabotage it. The best way to deal with the Inner Critic is to ignore her and keep writing. If yours is particularly bothersome and refuses to be ignored, try this exercise.

When you sit down to write, take an extra piece of paper and at the top write 'Negative Scratch Pad'. Each and every time a negative thought or judgement occurs, turn to your negative scratch pad and write it down.

I can't write
This is a joke – who do I think I am?
Everything I write is useless
I have no imagination
I'm boring
I'm sick of hearing myself say I'm boring…

At the end of the writing session feel free to rip up your scratch pad and throw it in the bin. Gradually, as your Inner Critic realizes just how little power she has, the negative, inhibiting, self-critical thoughts will dry up, leaving you more and more freedom to write from your core.

We have both found the practice of writing immensely enriching. It has given us a deeper sense of self as well as sharpened our senses to the world around us. Time and again writing has also been a personal form of therapy, guiding us from confusion and chaos towards clarity and a much deeper trust in life itself.

Chapter 4

Charisma – *the* beauty *of* energy

Charisma. It is a word of Greek origins which weaves magnetism, presence, energy and attraction into one magnificent tapestry. Charisma is the essence of good looks. And good looks matter. To maintain they do not is an absurd pretention. How you look and dress and move, what you wear (or opt not to wear), your make-up – all of these are *external* expressions of who you *are*. They are not trivial things, separate from you and without meaning. Each is just as important as how you think and eat and how well you honour your inner values.

One of the first signs of emotional disturbance in a woman is a neglect of the way she looks. Numerous psychological studies attest to the power that a good haircut, make-up and daily skin care have in enhancing self-esteem and alleviating emotional symptoms in depressed, anxious or troubled people. External self-neglect is just as energy-wasting and self-destructive as living by somebody else's rules or trying to survive on plastic food. Greasy hair and a pullover that carries traces of last Tuesday's lunch simply don't make it.

Manbait? No sir!

Many staunch feminists expound the belief that if a woman cares about external things she is undermining female power by allowing herself to be treated as a decorative sexual object. Although we are completely at one with the goals of the feminist movement when it comes to empowering political thought and action and securing equal pay, we believe there are two huge flaws in such an argument. The first is the belief that a woman only takes care over her appearance to attract a man. It is a notion we find insulting. We care about how we look because we care about ourselves. In a world in which, by some weird set of circumstances, all men disappeared, we would take just as much care.

The second, and far more important flaw to such an argument, lies in its misplaced dismissal of the real power and value of female sexuality. So important is its expression (in whatever form it takes) to every woman committed to the process of learning to live in the fullness of her being that to deny your sexuality would be to encase yourself in a straitjacket just as restricting as the woman-as-sex-symbol nonsense. A non-sexual woman is a woman cut off from the instinctual part of her nature – a woman who only allows herself to be half alive. To live from your core is to celebrate your wholeness and individuality *internally* and *externally*.

There are lots of ways of approaching good looks. You can read the glossy magazines then rush out to buy the latest eyeshadows. You can copy what looks good on somebody else and hope for the best. You can lament your big nose or sagging breasts and head for the nearest plastic surgeon. All well and good if that is what you fancy. But we think there is a better and far more empowering way: opt for charisma. It is the most dynamic, authentic and amusing approach of all.

Go for charisma

The word charisma literally means 'talent, grace, a favour especially vouchsafed by God'. The charisma approach to good looks focuses not so much on specifics as on the overall impression you create – an expression of your personal and idiosyncratic feeling for who you are and what looks best on you. This is something of far greater value than a docile conformity to conventional notions about fashion and beauty. The charisma approach to good looks is bold, assertive and often witty. And, contrary to popular opinion, it is not the exclusive province of the special elect – women with perfect size 10 bodies and not a wrinkle on their faces. Far from it. Charisma is ageless. It exists in every culture. It is the icing on the endless-energy cake – the *external* expression of your unique authenticity which gives you panache, boldness and humour and transforms physical limitations like wide hips or giraffe necks into assets. It can make a wonderful *statement* out of a nose that by conventional standards is too big. It makes you stand out in a crowd. Developing charisma of your own can not only be a lot of fun and have a dazzling effect on your outside world, it can even empower you to live more and more from your core.

Affirming what's authentic

What gives you charisma? The Chanel suit you wear? The car you drive? The way you have been taught to use your body or speak your words? Not really. For stylish or charming as these things may be, they are often chosen without any consideration of whether or not they have a connection with the individuality of the woman who wears them.

It is rather like hanging Christmas baubles on a willow tree. As such they offer little more than the appearance of charisma. And like pastiche, appearances never deceive a discerning eye.

Charisma – the real McCoy – has certain characteristics. Expansiveness, for instance, and joy, creativity and authenticity. The more you trust yourself and allow your own brand of energy to flow from within, the more your own charisma develops naturally. It works the other way round too. The more fun you have exploring different modes of self-expression using colour, clothes and make-up, as well as different female archetypes, the more you call forth your own brand of this energy of beauty. Then the Chanel suit or the recycled dress from Oxfam, or the wild rastafarian dreadlocks you decide to wear, take on a whole new flavour. You begin to use them not as status badges of acceptability or rebellion but for the enjoyment and aesthetic pleasure they bring. They become no more than another means of expressing whatever you want to express about yourself. Once this begins to happen you can break through forever the barrier of exploitation which is so destructive to a woman's sense of personal value and which operates so heavily in our commercial society. Developing your own charisma is first a question of acknowledging that how you look matters. Secondly you need to make time to care for yourself and to explore who you are. Finally you have to rediscover the art of play.

Your unique nature can be expressed in a myriad of ways from the most simple and playful to the most profound: in the colours you like best, in the way you choose to wear your hair and the kind of make-up you use as well as how you think and talk, and in the deep values you embody, even in the dreams you dream and in the things you do and make whether they be creations of art, intellectual or physical feats, or your simple day-to-day ways of being. That is why, at its essence, charisma is both disarmingly simple and immeasurably complex – neither more nor less than living day by day from a full and honest outpouring of your individuality – that spirit which is unique to you.

Self-expression or self-indulgence

It is a funny thing about self-expression. We in the Anglo Saxon world tend to think of it as something self-indulgent or self-obsessive. We have been brought up in a culture that affirms the value of altruism and insists that one should forget oneself in constant service and self-sacrifice to others. This is particularly true of women. Many of us spend our whole lives in one way or another denying our own needs and worrying about others, or following a career path which society's values (not one's own) have imposed upon us. Then we wake up at the age of 45 to find that we feel lost and empty, and that life is without meaning.

The truth is that at the heart of serving others, as well as at the core of nurturing life, lies the need to live fully as you are. For you can bring to others the full impact of your aliveness through your beauty, intellect, enthusiasm, compassion, creativity, fun and joy only when you actually have access to it yourself. This is why the pathway towards endless energy asks that you explore such personal and supposedly self-indulgent things as the kind of eyeshadow you wear or how best to look after your skin and how to make yourself look and feel more beautiful.

Only when the pursuit of beauty becomes a thing *apart* from the expression of your individual nature does it go all wrong. This is because beauty, treated only as an external, has sad repercussions for your own sense of self-worth. Like the old mechanistic worldview which has blinded us to what we have been doing to our planet, it can imprison you within false images and feelings of inadequacy that make it impossible to live creatively or bring the joy of your own unique energy to those around you.

Contacting your unique spirit, coming to respect it, and having the courage to live from it, in all of its many manifestations, is what developing charisma is all about. Sometimes challenging, frequently exciting, this process can be a lot of fun too. As it takes place the externals in your life – the clothes and make-up, the way you move and how you relate to your world, cease to be arbitrary or things you pick up with uncertainty to carry around with you or to hide behind. Instead they develop and unfold beautifully and mysteriously – almost organically – from within, as ever more potent expressions of who you are.

Workbook *for* Charisma – *The* beauty *of* energy

Let's get down to the nuts and bolts of charisma – the seemingly superficial trimmings such as make-up, hairstyle and fashion which can help you explore who you are and feel good about yourself. As you will discover, when you select these trimmings and trappings from core impulses and desires the results are anything *but* superficial.

The first step in developing your own brand of charisma is to get to know and make friends with the many facets of yourself. Each facet is like a character just itching for the chance to play a role in your life. When you encourage your characters to find expression, your reward is not only a great deal of pleasure and fun but an abundance of core energy.

Charisma detectors

The following steps can reveal clues to characters inside you who carry energy for you. Answer each question as fully as you can in your journal. Also make a note of any feelings (good or bad) that come up as you do the exercise. You might like to work with a friend, one of you asking the questions and noting down the answers while the other allows her fantasies to run free. Whether you work with a friend or on your own, let yourself *play* at it. Although the issues that arise are important, exploring charisma above all means having fun.

Choose a photograph

Find a photograph of yourself that you like. (For some this may not be easy, but you can at least find a photo that you prefer to others.) Ask yourself why you have chosen this picture. What do you like about the person you see? What qualities does she have? How is the person in the photo the same as, and how is she different from, the person you feel yourself to be now?

Scan your wardrobe

Make a note of any item or items of your wardrobe that you really love, things you feel good in – it could be a dress or a pair of shoes. (It could be something from your past or even something that you once borrowed.) Now ask yourself what it is you like about this particular thing. What qualities does it express? How does it make you feel? What image/character does it suggest?

Pick your accessories

Make a note of accessories, past, present or future, that you particularly like. Include jewellery, scarves, belts, hats, gloves, glasses, the lot. What is it about the accessory that you like? What does it remind you of? What part of you does it express?

How about your hair?

Ask yourself what was your favourite haircut or hairstyle/hair colour? Why did you like it? How did it make you feel? What aspect of you did it express?

What is your look?

Ask yourself is there an item of make-up that you particularly like? Or more than one? What do you like about the way that make-up makes you feel? What part of you does it help to express?

Write into life

If one or more of your characters is particularly exciting, get to know her by writing her into existence. Describe her as fully as you can. What does she wear? What is her hair like? Her make-up? Her nails? How does she move? Where does she go? What does she do? How does she speak? What does she say? What does she like and hate?

Although simple, this exercise is powerful and can evoke a lot of different feelings, thoughts and memories. Whatever comes up for you, acknowledge it by writing it down, no matter how insignificant or stupid it may seem. Anything can be a clue to helping your charisma unfold from the core. Commonly women feel a sense of hopelessness and longing. They may have an image of a character who seems to be everything they feel they are not. Then, instead of inspiring them, the image over-whelms them. If this is the case, remember that your character carries energy for you because she reflects an important part of you. No matter how far away from the-you-which-you-know she may seem, you can begin to live her right now. Obviously if your character is a waif-like wood nymph and you are 3 stone overweight it will take time to adjust this difference. Nevertheless it may be that by rearranging your hair or wearing a colour that the wood nymph would wear you can begin to draw upon her as an inspiration and start to tap into her quality of energy. Let these images inspire not discourage you. The best way to deal with a sense of discouragement in the face of anything that seems impossible is to begin by making a tiny step in the direction you want to go. We have learnt over and over that the way to climb a mountain (either physical or metaphorical) is just to put one foot in front of the other.

In exploring charisma it can be very freeing to break the rules and try something completely new. For instance, if you always wear make-up to work, dare one day to go completely bare faced. Leslie frequently used to go to work as the health and beauty editor of a magazine, wearing no make-up. She found it immensely freeing to break the rules and discovered it gave her a fresh sense of herself.

Go wild – dress up

Remember as a little girl what fun it was to dress up? Remember the thrill of wearing high heels and lipstick? Rediscover the joy of playing dressing-up games. It's a great way to free yourself from convention and the limitations of how you feel you 'should' look. Choose a character for inspiration that is as different as possible from the way you ordinarily see your-self. Then go wild: paint your face, restyle your hair or put a colour rinse on it, dress up in something you wouldn't normally dare wear, add scarves, beads, bangles, feathers – whatever enhances your look. What have you discovered about yourself in the process?

Your dressing table

One of the most transformative exercises for any woman can be making an altar to honour her inner and outer beauty. When you create a place and a space in time in which to celebrate and enhance your looks, you give yourself credit and a new sense of self-worth. You also access power and energy you didn't know you had.

Find a suitable place

Choose a place you like in your bedroom (or perhaps in your bathroom if it is large enough).

Make this space a priority by moving anything unnecessary out of the way. Ideally the place should have a good source of natural and artificial light (for applying make-up or styling your hair – day or night), and be near an electricity socket to plug in hairdryers and other electrical equipment.

Making a dressing table

If you have a dressing table that you like – great. If not, you can make one from a table with a stand-up mirror or, failing a table, even an upturned orange crate covered with a pretty cloth. In addition to the stand-up mirror, a hand mirror is useful to see the back of your head or different angles of your face.

Create your decor

Gather together any objects that inspire you – a lace handkerchief on which to place things, a few pebbles or shells, a candle – whatever you find beautiful. Find the photograph of yourself which you particularly liked from the first exercise and frame it to place on your dressing table. If you have a favourite inspiring quotation or a picture or postcard that pleases you, add that. You can even use a picture cut out of a magazine for inspiration. (Ask yourself what it is about the picture that you like and what quality in *you* it reflects.)

Organize your stuff

Find baskets or boxes in which to organize your make-up, hair things, face and body-care products, jewellery, etc. If you have dressing-table drawers, line them with attractive paper or material. If you lack drawer space, keep your things in boxes of different shapes and sizes. Hat boxes are great for bulky things like hair rollers. We also like to cover old shoe boxes with wrapping paper or wallpaper to make pretty containers. Arrange your items in such a way that they are easily accessible and fun to use – for instance stand brushes and eye/lip pencils upright in a cylindrical container.

Junk the junk

Sort through your beauty things and get rid of *everything* that isn't useful and doesn't inspire you. If you can't bring yourself to throw or give things away, such as a piece of jewellery you were given that you never wear but can't bear to part with, put the items away in a cupboard so your dressing table holds only the things you like best.

As you sort through your belongings make a list of anything you need that you don't have, such as the right colour blusher, or some tissues instead of the toilet roll you are making do with for blotting your lips. Make an effort to get the missing items as soon as possible.

Make offerings

Gather together all the things you need to enhance your beauty such as face and body treats (see p.37 for suggestions). Imbue the objects with power by offering them to your core characters. For instance, if there is an Amazon in you seeking expression you might encourage her by choosing a self-massage instrument for improving muscle tone or honour her with a postcard of the goddess Artemis.

We like to keep fresh flowers on our dressing tables. They are a symbol of beauty. And, because they need to be renewed, they remind you to honour the beauty within you.

Take as much time as you need to arrange your dressing table to your liking. Notice any feelings that arise as you organize things. One common feeling is guilt: 'I shouldn't be spending so much time on myself' or 'I can't really justify doing this when I have so many more important things to do.' Whatever feelings come up, make a note of them in your journal and no matter how guilty you feel or how unjustified, do it anyway! Some women who have done this exercise with us have found it had a profound effect on them. Rather like deep meditation it brought to the surface all sorts of revelations about themselves that had little to do with face creams and lipsticks.

Some of Leslie's favourite dressing table items have turned out to be:
- **A crumbling eighteenth-century sconce** above the dressing table decorated with gold leaf and hung with a Japanese and a Venetian mask: 'The sconce reminds me of the fun of fantasy of Cocteau's *Beauty and the Beast*.'
- **A hat box filled with different coloured ribbons:** 'Ribbons, for me, are a symbol of womanhood. I draw inspiration from all the colours. I like to wear them in my hair. It's a way of decorating myself with colour in the way that tribal women or peasants do.'
- **A basket with two hairdryers plugged in:** 'I find drying my hair so boring that I like to get it over with quickly by using two hairdryers at once. I keep them

easily accessible in a round basket beneath my dressing table so that getting dressed after my morning run and shower takes as little time as possible.'

● **The bleached vertebrae of a sheep:** 'Given to me years ago by my eldest son, it reminds me of how impermanent outer beauty is and helps me affirm the beauty of my own and other women's spirit.'

And Susannah's:

● **A basket full of make-up goodies:** 'I keep my essential make-up items in a beautiful basket decorated with a bow and feathers. The basket is inviting and easy to dip into whenever I need a make-up boost. I keep an "experimental box" with more outlandish make-up, hair accessories, etc. for when I'm feeling adventurous.

● **A collection of rocks and shells:** 'I have always found great beauty and inspiration from the sea. My rocks and shells are purely for decoration and yet arranging them in pleasing ways helps me to feel rearranged too.'

● **Lots of small perfume bottles:** 'I love pretty perfume bottles and enjoy exploring different characters in myself by wearing different fragrances. I collect perfume samples for travelling and carrying around. An advantage to small bottles is that you use perfume up before it has a chance to go off. Leslie has another approach... "Buy large bottles and use it lavishly!"'

Face and body treats

Keep a selection of face and body treats on your dressing table to encourage you to pamper yourself. Here are some suggestions.

Beauty in a capsule

Flaxseed oil or Evening Primrose oil in capsule form makes an ideal daily or weekly face treat. After cleansing your skin, simply pierce a capsule with a pin and spread the contents over your face. After 30 minutes tissue off any excess oil that hasn't been absorbed (see Resources, p.136).

Spot fix

We have found a good-quality pure Tea Tree oil to be helpful for almost any skin problem – from acne to an allergic rash. Apply the oil sparingly to the problem area 3 times a day until it clears.

Facial sauna treat

Keep a small bottle of German or Roman Chamomile essential oil on your dressing table to remind yourself to have a facial sauna once a week. Chamomile makes a wonderful sauna whether your skin is dry or oily. Add a few drops of the oil to a basin of boiling water. Hold a towel over your head to create a tent and keep your face as close to the steaming water as is comfortable for 5 minutes. Rinse your skin in warm water and rub an ice cube across it as a toner, then moisturize.

Anti-wrinkle tablets

An exciting discovery in internal cosmetics is the use of nutritional supplements of fish cartilage and marine extracts. It is the *only* naturopathic formula ever double-blind tested in hospitals and reported in international medical journals. It supports the biochemical processes in your skin that produce new elastin and new collagen, enabling them to work in an optimal way. The result is smoother, firmer, younger-looking skin (see Resources, p.137).

Massage tools

There are some wonderful massage tools that can help tone the body and shift cellulite deposits. The simplest is a dry-skin brush or hemp glove which can be used all over the body before your shower or bath (see p.78 for instructions.) There are also some superb commercial self-massage implements which are designed to help eliminate cellulite when used in conjunction with a cream or oil (see Resources, p.136).

Thirsty skin treat

As an all-over body moisturizer it's hard to beat pure cold-pressed flaxseed oil, a unique balance of linoleic and linolenic fatty acids. It makes your skin more beautiful on the surface. It is also readily absorbed and energizes cellular activity which helps prevent lumps and bumps. To preserve its freshness you *must* keep it in the refrigerator rather than on your dressing table. After a bath or shower spread it over your skin, concentrating on any dry, rough patches.

If you find you can't get flaxseed oil, try pure sesame or almond oil instead. Both of these can also double as massage oils. For a soothing or relaxing massage, add a few drops of geranium essential oil to 50 ml of the flaxseed oil. Alternatively, for an invigorating massage, use a few drops of peppermint essential oil instead.

Your make-up kit

Here are some items we find useful in a basic make-up kit at our dressing table or when travelling. You might like to use it as a guideline to create your own: foundation, eyebrow pencil, eyebrow brush, eyeliner pencil(s), eyeshadow(s), mascara, eyelash curler, blusher, lipcolour, lip pencil, lip salve or gloss, eye drops, (a small tube of toothpaste and a toothbrush for travelling), nail file, facial or lip tissues.

Foundation

Choose a colour as close as possible to your natural skin tone. Trying to add colour or a tan with foundation rarely looks good – leave that job to your blusher.

Tips: mature skins tend to be dry and are therefore best suited to a liquid foundation. For younger or oily skin a compact foundation is ideal and can be used to smooth out the complexion in specific areas where needed.

Brow tools

Brows: choose a colour to match your brows in order to accentuate their shape and fill in any gaps.

Tips: we particularly like automatic pencils because they never get blunt. Feather the colour on against the direction of hair growth and then brush the brows into shape. Eyebrow colour gives a face definition – especially helpful for those with very light hair. For a clean line, tweeze any straggly hairs away from under the brow. As we get older, our body hair becomes thinner. Taking a supplement of organic silica (about 800 to 1200mg per day, see Resources, p.137) can help keep your eyebrows and lashes full.

Eyeliner

Choose a colour which accentuates the colour of your eyes rather than competing with it. A bright blue crayon, for example, will only make blue eyes look dull by comparison. Instead, try soft lilac, heather, taupe, grey, neutral brown, grey/blue or grey green. It's nice to use two complementary shades – a lighter one beneath the lower lashes and a darker one above the upper. Make sure your crayon is gentle and soft.

Tips: apply the colour(s) from the centre of the upper and lower lids outwards, blending to an angle at the outer corner of the eye. Your eye crayon can double for shadow. Make a palette from the back of your hand and mix the crayon together with a little moisturizer or liquid foundation then apply to the crease of your eye socket and blend out and up.

Eyeshadow

As with your eyeliner, choose colours that bring out the beauty of your eyes. Matt colours in earth tones work better than bright glittery ones.

Tips: usually two eye colours are enough – a lighter one such as a golden cream or pale apricot for highlighting under the brow and on the lid and a darker shade such as a taupe or soft brown for emphasizing the eye socket. If your eyes are prominent use the darker shade on the lid and keep the highlighter for the brow bone and inner corner of the lid only.

Eyelash gear

Choose mascara to suit your hair colour: black or charcoal for dark hair, auburn or grey for red heads and brown or grey for blondes.

Tips: even though we are both spontaneous criers, we always prefer non-waterproof mascara. The waterproof variety is difficult to remove and when it does run is impossible to shift. We swear by eyelash curlers. They make your lashes look twice as long and thick. Use the curler on your upper lashes for a few seconds before applying your mascara. Then apply the mascara to the top and underside of the upper lashes and to the lower lashes if desired. For special occasions try this discreet falsie trick. Trim false eyelashes to about one third of their length and apply them to the outer edges of your upper lashes. Apply mascara to blend with your natural lashes. These shortie lashes are much easier to manipulate and make your eyes look beautifully doe-like.

Blusher

As with eye colour, go easy on the glittery stuff. Preferably choose a matt colour to match your natural blush. The colour of the inside of your mouth is a good guideline. Older women should choose their shade particularly carefully to give a natural-looking glow – pastel melon or peach are better than fuchsia pink or burgundy. Cream blushers often have better staying power than powders.

Tips: apply blusher over your cheek bones tapering towards the temples. We find the brushes in compacts are usually too small and prefer a large wedge-shaped brush. The right shade of blusher can also be used as eyeshadow: apply to the eye socket as well as the cheeks and chin or your décolleté to make even the most tired face look bright and well.

Lip colour

Finding your ideal lip colour is rather like being a surfer waiting for the perfect wave – you wonder if it actually exists. A good solution is to use one colour over another to create your own blend.

Tips: we like to line our lips first with a tone just *slightly* darker than our natural colour – a neutral sepia shade for instance – and then fill it in with a lip colour, such as a terracotta or beigey pink, or simply a gloss or salve. Here are a few tricks we find useful.

A clear or gold lip gloss applied to the lower lip gives the mouth warmth. For a sexy pout use this Hollywood trick: apply a darker lip colour to the upper lip and a lighter one to the lower. For staying power apply your lipstick once, then blot and apply a second layer. To avoid leakage of colour into the cracks around your mouth prepare a good base by applying foundation first. Then blot your lips, dust with powder and apply your lip colour. If you are wearing a strong colour, outline the outer edge of your lips with a skin-coloured pencil to keep your lipstick from spreading.

Scoop out the ends of your favourite old lipsticks and add the bits to a small flat tin (such as those used for mints or pills). Melt the lip colours down with the help of a candle or lighter and mix well to create an original shade. Apply the lip colour with a lip brush or with your finger.

Play with perfume

Fragrances have a powerful ability to evoke feelings and impressions. The perfume you choose, like your clothes and make-up, makes a strong statement about who you are. It's fun to create a perfume wardrobe so that you can choose a fragrance to suit your mood. You can also use scent to draw out a character within you that needs encouragement.

Women with a highly developed sense of smell tend to choose scents as an expression not of their outer personality but rather of one or more of their inner, core characters. For instance, a sexually assured and outgoing business woman (once she has moved beyond the straitjacket of brand-name snobbery) will often choose a light and delicate floral while her shy and introverted sister will be more likely to opt for a heavy seductive oriental. What a well-chosen perfume should do is allow you to explore whatever quality (extroverted, introverted, dreamy, stable, sensuous or clear) you wish to develop further at any particular time. Most perfumes fall into 4 families. Here is a guide to these families and to the type of statement that each one makes.

The feminine florals

These scents express undeniable femininity, great for the Romantic, the English Rose, the Princess, the Country Lady, the Medieval Maiden or the Nature Spirit. They are made from fragrant blossoms and rely heavily on jasmine, tuberose, rose and gardenia. Florals are delightful worn singly or in a blend. Examples of blends include: *Fiji* by Guy Laroche, *Joy* by Jean Patou, Nina Ricci's *L'Air du Temps*, *Oscar de la Renta*, Lagerfeld's *Chloé*, Guerlain's *Jardin de Bagatelle*, *Amarige* by Givenchy, *Trésor* by Lancôme, *Paris* by Yves St Laurent, *Kenzo*, Elizabeth Arden's *Blue Grass*, *Joseph*, Calvin Klein's *Eternity* and *Escape*, *Dune* by Christian Dior (floral-oceanic), *Safari* by Ralph Lauren and *Feminité du Bois* by Shiseido.

The mysterious orientals

Rich, sultry scents for the overtly seductive woman who likes to be noticed: the Seductress, the Witch, the Gypsy and the Earth Goddess. Made from Eastern woods and spices, these fragrances are often tempered with the nostalgic odour of vanilla or spiked with spice. They are great when you are feeling bold, or bring out the seductress in you when you feel timid. Traditional orientals include: Estée Lauder's *Youth Dew*, *Cinnabar* and *SpellBound* (a floral-oriental), Guerlain's *Shalimar*, *Ysatis* by Givenchy (semi-oriental), *Dioressence*, Lancôme's *Magie Noire*, *Opium* by Yves St Laurent, *Obsession* by Calvin Klein, *Loulou* by Cacharel, *Poison* by Dior, or *Bijan Oscar de la Renta*.

Cool greens

These fragrances give an impression of freedom. They offer swift-moving, clear-thinking independence for the Shaman, the Amazon, the Athlete, the Gamine and the Anarchist. They are fresh, cool and uplifting – ideal for expressing (or discovering) the athlete within. The green family of scents relies on aromatic woods such as cedar and sandalwood, mosses, ferns and grasses for its unique character. Classic greens include: Balmain's *Vent Vert*, Yves St Laurent's 'Y', Estée Lauder's *Alliage*, *Chanel No. 19*, *Givenchy III*, *Diorissimo* by Christian Dior, Cacharel's *Anaïs Anaïs*, *Lauren* by Ralph Lauren and *Giò* by Giorgio Armani.

Aldehydics

This fragrance group expresses a rich and modern sophistication, wonderful for the Glitzy Power-Broker, the Sophisticated Lady and the Executive. The aldehydics are particularly compatible with the cultural and intellectual excitement of city life. Based on a chemical group known as the aldehydes which gives them their unmistakable power, the aldehydics are also characterized by a rich floral quality including such notes as citrus, jasmine, rose and geranium, as well as musk. Examples include: *Chanel No. 5*, *Diorama*, *Arpège* by Lanvin, *Farouche* by Nina Ricci, *Calandre* by Paco Rabanne, *Chamade* and *Samsara* by Guerlain, Hermes' *Calèche*, Yves St Laurent's *Rive Gauche*, Estée Lauder's *White Linen*, *Madame Rochas* and *Byzance* by Rochas, Givenchy's *L'Interdit*, *Enigma* by Charles of the Ritz and *Je Reviens* by Worth.

Buying a fragrance

Most of us make the mistake of buying a perfume to suit what we think is our image. And following the advertiser's images doesn't work because fragrance is too personal so we end up looking at 6 different bottles on the dressing table, none of which we want to wear. For you to enjoy the fragrance you wear it must be chosen by instinct – because it feels good – not by intellect. Here are some of the practicalities to consider when perfume buying:

● Try no more than 5 perfumes at any one time and only 2 or 3 if they are similar.

● Spread the samples as far apart as possible on your arms so the smells don't mix.

● Allow the perfume enough time to develop on your skin before buying it.

● Don't just buy a perfume because it smells good on someone else. The condition of your skin, your diet and your own body odour will alter the character of a perfume.

● Department store perfume halls are not ideal for trying out scents – there are just too many smells for your olfactory system to cope with. It is better to collect samples and try them at home.

● When you've found a fragrance you like, put it where your skin is warm and where there's a good circulation of blood. Behind the ears, under clothing or on pulse points are all wonderful places or, in the words of Coco Chanel, 'wherever you expect to be kissed'.

● Fragrance is an unabashed statement of yourself. Indulge your senses and enjoy finding the right one for you.

Your wardrobe

What woman hasn't at some point succumbed to the proverbial wail: 'I haven't got a thing to wear!'? Just as setting up a dressing table to honour your inner and outer beauty can bring you inspiration and a new sense of self-esteem, taking your wardrobe to task can give you a tremendous energy boost. By clearing out what doesn't work for you, you can see more clearly what does. As you do, it helps crystallize your sense of self. Then the cry of the wardrobe victim with nothing to wear, can empower you to find a solution.

Look through your wardrobe and remove any items of clothing which you don't wear. Ask yourself why..?

● Do the items need mending/cleaning? If so, don't put it off – you deserve to make the effort for yourself.

● Are the items too big or too small? If you have gained or lost weight, but you think your weight might change back again, store these items away in a box until they do fit. That way your wardrobe only contains the things that you can wear right now.

● Do you dislike the style or shape? the colour? the length? If you like an item, but it doesn't quite work, see if it's possible to adjust it so that it does. If you know you'll never get around to fixing/dyeing it – sacrifice it.

● Do you simply hate wearing some things? If so, allow yourself the freedom to give them away or throw them away – whichever is more appropriate.

Reorganize your clothes so what you have is accessible and getting dressed is fun. Make a list in your journal of any item of clothing or accessory that you feel you need but don't have. Bear in mind the needs of the characters within trying to find expression. Make an action plan for yourself to pick them up – new or secondhand according to your budget.

Part two

Taking Stock

Each journey has its pleasures and its perils and each traveller her strengths and her weaknesses.

It is in honouring the strengths and focusing clarity and kindness on the weaknesses that each of us makes her own passages to power.

Chapter 5

Weeding out *the* blockers *and* drainers

The seed of a plant, nestled into the earth, needs a good rich soil and plenty of light and water to thrive. So do you in your own way. And, as any good gardener knows, you have to pull out as many weeds as possible to help a tiny seedling develop into full flower. Weeds have two negative effects. First they drain energy, sapping the soil of goodness. Secondly they block energy by inhibiting growth. Their overgrowth in the flowerbed can mean too little space for the seedling to unfold. So it is with us. No woman can realize the full potential of her capacity for energy, health and good looks while she is struggling against too many *energy-drainers* and *energy blockers*.

Meet the energy-drainers

Our world is full of energy-drainers. Excessive noise in cities, environmental poisons in our air and our water, foods and chemicals that we come in contact with and to which (often unbeknownst to us) we may be sensitive or allergic – all these drain energy. Their presence in your life, particularly if you have a sensitive disposition, can undermine your vitality – lowering your immunity and making you susceptible not only to colds and flu but also to premature ageing and the development of degenerative conditions.

It might surprise you to learn that there are *internal* factors that can be just as energy wasting. Take a relationship which depends on you compromising your own values in a major way or changing yourself to suit what you think the other person wants you to be. When any woman goes against herself or forces herself to be hypocritical she squanders her core energy.

Wasting anxiety

Few emotions drain energy like anxiety. While you dash about (either physically or in your consciousness) feeling unsafe and unstable and trying like mad to make everything seem all right, you deplete your body and your creativity. Where there is anxiety there is a high level of electrical, electropositive magnetic activity and chemical acidity which affect the sympathetic nervous system and encourage feelings of fear, irritability, nausea and headache, as well as an inability to concentrate, muscle pain and insomnia. Even minor attacks of nervousness can dramatically undermine your work performance and make it almost impossible for you to enjoy yourself.

Anxiety is frequently related to food allergies. Re-aligning your diet can help. So can physical exercise which calms electrical and chemical overactivity, replacing it with a more balanced energy, which you can call on, and a feeling of mental and physical wellbeing.

Depression can be a big energy-drainer as well. It too often grows out of a biochemical imbalance. This could be caused, for example, by living on a diet of processed convenience foods which deplete your body of the minerals essential for its energy-transmitting pathways to function properly and for brain chemicals which keep your spirits high to be formed in adequate quantities. Sometimes depression develops as a result of blocked emotions which you may not even be aware you are feeling – like grief. Often depression is rather like an anger turned in on yourself to block you from doing harm to anyone else. In any case, once you feel depression, you get caught up in a vicious circle where your low-energy state only further feeds the negative state and vice versa. To break through and release the energy that has been blocked by depression you may need to examine your experience of depression carefully as well as change your lifestyle. More about how in chapter 8, Passage to Power.

Hapless habits

Habits can drain core energy too. Smoking for instance. In a biochemical way tobacco uses up nutrients like vitamin C, zinc and bioflavonoids which are necessary to preserve healthy wrinkle-free skin and to maintain the good circulation that brings oxygen to the organs and tissues all over your body. Because it is a form of addictive behaviour, smoking saps core energy in other ways too. It only helps to let off steam without positive payoffs. Like all addictive behaviour, smoking can mask deeper dissatisfactions and blockages to the full development of your seedpower by trapping you in vicious circles which lead you to feel more and more dead rather than more and more alive.

Good and bad energy

When you eat, your body breaks the food down chemically through digestion allowing you to absorb the nutrients into your cells and your blood. There it is turned into the building blocks of life and chemical energy, which is electromagnetic energy – the energy of life. All physical and mental energy in nature involves *electromagnetics*. Each of your cells has a positive and a negative field. All physical, emotional and mental events are brought about by chemical reactions triggered by electromagnetic impulses from the brain. Food is not the only source of life energy. The metabolism of food is supplemented by electromagnetic energy from the brain and from geomagnetic energy.

For a long time the biomagnetic aspects of living organisms were ignored because both biology and medicine tend to leave biophysics out of their discipline. Now, however, thanks to discoveries in quantum physics and biomagnetics, and to the development of many interesting diagnostic and treatment tools using magnetic energy like nuclear magnetic resonance (used to replace x-rays and cut out the danger of radiation) and diapulse instruments for the treatment of pain, a new awareness of the body not only as a chemical and physical phenomenon but as a biomagnetic one is emerging. It is an important area to know about when it comes to maximizing your own energy.

The body electric

As well as drawing energy from food, your body absorbs magnetic energy from the earth itself. Some animals such as sharks and certain insects appear to draw more energy from the earth's field than they do from the food they eat. The earth's natural pulsing frequency is 7.96 cycles per second – a frequency at which, as it happens, we thrive. Your body even takes in energy when you breathe. The oxygen in the air, is itself paramagnetic – that is, able to take a magnetic charge. It

---

WOMEN AND DEPRESSION

According to recent research, women are twice as susceptible to depression as men. One obvious factor is the female biological make-up with its hormonal cycles that contribute to mood swings. But there are also social factors. According to the American Psychological Association, the structure of our society, which tends to place women in more passive roles than men, creates a sense of impotence – making women more prone to dissatisfaction and depression. The APA's Task Force on Women and Depression also found that thirty-seven per cent of the women suffering from depression who were studied had been victims of significant physical or sexual abuse by the age of 21.

carries the earth's magnetic field into all the cells of your body within a few seconds.

There are many ways in which you can intensify the electromagnetic life energy on which your body and mind run. Exercising for instance. One of the laws of physics states that a liquid flowing through a magnetic field creates an electromotive force. In nature, where you have a waterfall you also have an abundance of electromagnetic energy created around it by the action of the water flowing through the earth's magnetic field. In the body this same phenomenon happens. During exercise blood and lymph flow freely and become an *internal* source of magnetic energy on which you thrive. Using alternately hot and cold water over the surface of your skin, as in many hydrotherapy techniques, also produces biomagnetic energy for you to use. Finally, and vitally important to high level health, so does sleep via the gentle movement of cerebral spinal fluid.

Electropollution and electroconfusion

All these energy-creating sources and mechanisms would be great if it weren't for the fact that our lifestyle with its electrical appliances, high-tension cables, televisions and VDUs produce an enormous amount of electromagnetic contamination and confusion. Your body thrives not on chaos but on *order*. Wherever you have an electrical appliance, wherever you have wiring in a house, you have electromagnetic fields. Things you use commonly such as hairdryers, toasters and radios all create fields of 50 to 60 cycles per second. This higher frequency fatigues the body's cells (which thrive on the earth's natural 7.96 cycles per second) and can deplete or disrupt your own biomagnetic energy. Couple this with the virtually ubiquitous radio waves from walkabout phones, radio and television transmitting equipment and radar in our atmosphere, and you realize that, since the middle of the twentieth century, we have all been living in the midst of an insidious new form of pollution which can not be seen or felt and yet which can challenge the human immune system profoundly and create both mental and physical disorder.

Robert O. Becker MD has twice been nominated for a Nobel prize for his work in regenerating bones using electromagnetic fields. Considered *the* expert in the English-speaking world on the effects of electromagnetism, he warns strongly against sleeping on or under an electric blanket. Becker has studied the incidence of birth defects in pregnant women who use electric blankets and compared them to women who do not. He found that there is a significantly higher incidence of birth defects in women who do. And this is true even if they only use it to heat the bed and then turn it off before getting in. (You need to unplug an electric blanket completely to be safe.) Becker also warns strongly against having an old microwave oven in your kitchen. If you do, you should have it checked periodically for leakage as there is no statutory control over the leakage of microwaves from these devices. Using one over a period of time, he says, may seriously undermine health.

Two other experts in the field – Nancy Wertheimer and Ed Leeper in the United States – discovered that children living in homes near overhead electrical high-current wires were twice as likely to die from cancer as those who didn't. Although as yet there is little public awareness of it, electromagnetic pollution is a very real energy-drainer. Look at your own home and workplace and see what you can do to minimize it in your life.

Under the weather

Next time you feel out of sorts and somebody suggests it might be the weather, don't scoff. It too can drain energy. Age-old beliefs that 'ill winds' bring sickness, odd behaviour and general misery have been well supported by studies from all over the world correlating weather changes with such phenomena as suicide rates, crimes and various illnesses. In some people, the absence of light entering the eyes in winter or when time is constantly spent indoors results in extreme shifts in levels of melatonin – an important brain chemical which influences mood. This can lead to a condition known as Seasonal Affective Disorder or SAD where your energy seems to drain away and you get depressed or suffer disturbances in sleep and appetite. The remedy? Try exposing yourself to plenty of full-spectrum light *artificially*. Next time you replace a lighting fixture in your home or buy a desk lamp, go for one which uses full spectrum tubes instead of tungsten bulbs. Studies have shown that exposing SAD sufferers to full-spectrum lighting for several hours a day lifted the spirits of sixty to eighty per cent of those tested.

Another way in which the weather can drain energy is when there is an absence of negatively charged ions in the atmosphere. This can be the result of ill winds blowing, such as the Foehn in the Alps, the Sharav in the Middle East or the Chinook in America's

Rocky Mountains. Our modern concrete office buildings, furnished with synthetic materials and artificial air-conditioning, also lack negatively charged air ions. If you work in such an environment speak to your boss about how much he can decrease absenteeism amongst his employees by installing air purifiers and ionizers.

Confront the energy-blockers

Unlike the drainers which sap your energy, what we call the energy-blockers operate at a deeper level. They are things which seem to build walls around your core, hiding from you the very fact that your own deep energy resources exist, or which prevent you from building bridges with your external world. On an emotional and spiritual level these energy-blockers include an out-of-date or inappropriate worldview which prevents you from looking at your life and your future in a positive way, or false notions about yourself that make you feel isolated from the people with whom you live and work.

Energy-blockers, on a physical level, can be factors in your lifestyle that prevent the body's metabolic pathways involved in the production of energy from working efficiently. Such things include not getting enough exercise, living on a diet of processed foods or eating too much sugar. Over a period of time all three deplete your body of essential minerals and trace elements needed by enzymes to produce energy at a cellular level. To access your full share of energy in every area of your life you need to toss out these energy-blockers and replace them with energy-enhancing ways of using your body (see Chapters 9 and 10).

Resentment, too, can be an enormous energy-blocker. Anger immediately felt and expressed keeps energy flowing. Think of when you were a child and you got angry at a friend. It was quick to come and quick to pass so you could get on with whatever you both were doing. As adults we tend to swallow our anger, turning it into resentment.

Fear can also block energy. In a measurable physical way it freezes you into inactivity and makes all things seem impossible. Chronic fear, usually unconscious, can lead you to make the wrong choices because you feel the need continually to compromise on fundamental issues such as what you really want and particularly value.

So can negative feedback loops. When you feel low in energy you tend to attract energy-drainers which in turn attract other energy-drainers and before you know it you find yourself caught up in a negative feedback loop. You feel helpless – a victim of circumstances over which you have no power – and you lack the energy or the incentive to break out of the loop.

The energy-drainer scenario

A woman is in a job which she hates. She feels unmotivated and resentful (inner energy-drainers). After work she goes out to drink (alcohol-addiction drainer). Sometimes she drinks too much and this creates friction with her husband (relationship energy-drainer). She feels bad about herself as a result of arguing (emotional energy-drainer). Her poor self-image leads her not to care for herself (poor self-esteem energy-drainer). She eats badly (biochemical energy-drainer). She feels worse and suffers depression. Nothing in her life seems to work and she has nothing to look forward to…

You see the pattern. She is stuck in a rut. The energy-drainers have stolen her personal power and she can only see everything in the worst light.

Now let's look at the flip side. Energy-enhancers tend to attract other energy-enhancers, creating positive feedback loops and making you feel empowered and in control of your life. Compare the following situation with the previous sketch.

The energy-enhancer scenario

A woman is in a job which she hates. She discovers an inspiring exercise class (physical energy-booster). The class makes her feel good about herself and inspires her to eat better (biochemical booster). She loses a few pounds, feels better in her body and begins to dress in a more flattering way (self-esteem booster). She meets some new friends whose company she really enjoys (relationship booster). As her self-esteem increases, the people she works with begin to appreciate her more. Her job becomes more enjoyable (work booster). She feels excited about her life and confident about looking for a new job, something she will really love.

Identifying your own blockers and drainers, and making the choice to let go of even one or two, sows the seed for more positive feedback loops in your life. It is an important step to take in accessing more core energy and developing your personal power. Sometimes even awareness itself is enough to get the ball rolling.

Chapter 5
Workbook

Workbook *for* Weeding *out* *the* blockers *and* drainers

To weed out the energy-drainers and blockers from your life you first need to become aware of which ones are affecting you. In the charts on pp.46-48 you'll find many of the common outer and inner drainers, as well as useful hints on how to go about countering them. We don't suggest that you attempt to rid yourself of them all in one fell swoop. Rather, choose one or two that you think are particularly relevant to you. Make a note of them in your journal and decide to work towards eliminating them.

The process may be a gradual one. If, for instance, you decide to get rid of the convenience foods drainer, the process of learning to eat in a better way could take several months. Or the drainer you decide to counter could involve outside help from a friend, a self-help group or a professional expert. Some of the energy drainers – what we call The Sneaky Inner Drainers – are the result of the negative beliefs and feelings that one often harbours. After the charts you will find help in how to identify such drainers, as well as exercises that can enable you to free yourself of them. The important step in weeding out any blocker and drainer is making the decision to do so. This act in itself begins the process of drawing to you the information, people and power you need to carry out the change. There is a saying from Goethe which both of us like very much and which expresses the power of making a choice which is the beginning of creating what you want. It goes like this:
Whatever you can do or dream you can do, begin it. Boldness has genius, power and magic in it. Begin it now.

THE OUTER ENERGY-DRAINER
Energy-drainer/blocker
Electromagnetic Pollution
Heavy Metal Pollution: i.e. from lead, aluminium, mercury, cadmium
Weather
Office Pollution
Convenience Foods
Pesticides and Herbicides
Addictions
Overeating
Crash Dieting
Sedentary Lifestyle

Where is it found? What are the symptoms?	Helpful hints
Caused by static from electrical appliances, VDUs, TV, radio and portable phones, microwave ovens, electrical dial-face clocks. Results in mental and emotional confusion and hormonal imbalance.	Don't use electric blankets. Unplug TV at night. Sit 3 feet away from a VDU and 6 feet from TV. Get rid of your microwave. Sleep on magnetic bed.
Lead from car and industrial fumes, water from lead pipes. Cooking with aluminium pots, drinking orange juice packed in aluminium-lined boxes, using certain anti-perspirants. Mercury from tinned tuna and amalgam dental fillings. Heavy metals interfere with energy-producing enzymes in the body, leading to fatigue and mental/physical disorders.	Replace aluminium cooking pots/kettles. Drink spring water such as Volvic. Use sea algae supplements and add seaweed to soups and salads to chelate and eliminate the metals. Eat apples (pectin helps bind and remove heavy metals from the body).
Unusual winds and shifting barometric pressure cause depletion in negative ions resulting in depression, fatigue, irritable behaviour. Insufficient light during the winter months causes SAD (see p.44).	Use an ionizer in the room in which you work and by your bed at night (see Resources, p.137). Consider full-spectrum lighting (see Resources, p.136).
Concrete buildings, plastic furniture and synthetic decor deplete negative ions. Stale air recycled through conditioning and heating systems contains bacteria which challenge the immune system. Fluorescent lighting disturbs the nervous system, photocopier and printer chemicals can cause symptoms.	Use ionizers and replace fluorescent strip lights with full-spectrum ones. Keep photocopiers and printers in a room separate from the one in which you work. Take a break from your VDU for a few minutes every hour. Use radiation control screens.
Processed foods contain junk fats, refined flour and sugar, as well as artificial additives, flavourings and preservatives, which provoke biochemical chaos and can result in mental, physical symptoms.	Buy foods that are as close as possible to their natural state. Eat a good portion of your food raw. Go organic.
Chemically grown fruits, vegetables and cereals replete with toxic chemicals can deplete nutrients, disrupt enzyme reactions and pollute the body.	Buy organic. When you can't, after washing fruits and vegetables, soak for 20 minutes in a pan of water with 2 tablespoons of 10 volume H_2O_2.
Addictions to substances such as cigarettes, narcotics, alcohol, chocolate, sugar or caffeine upset the body's metabolic balance, depleting it of essential nutrients and leading to chronic fatigue.	Acknowledge your cravings as an addiction (see Chapter 6 for help).
Eating more than your body needs stresses the digestive system, depleting enzymes so that foods are badly broken down and poorly absorbed – deficiencies and chronic fatigue can result.	Eliminate cravings and false hunger by getting rid of junk foods and combining your foods well (see Chapter 9 for help). Look out for food allergies.
Fad diets are poorly balanced and deplete the body of vital nutrients, often resulting in fatigue and deficiency diseases such as anaemia. They also make you fat and flabby as you regain the weight you lost.	Look to a high-raw well-combined way of eating (see Chapter 9 for help) and find a form of exercise that inspires you if you want to shed excess fat.
Undermines your body's potential to produce electromagnetic energy and can result in calcium and magnesium being leeched from your bones, nails and hair, weakening them.	Get physical by walking briskly in comfortable shoes for 30 minutes a day, or dance, or swim, or run, and see how quickly you gain energy.

THE INNER ENERGY-DRAINERS AND BLOCKERS

Energy-drainer/ blocker	Where is it found? What are the symptoms?	Helpful hints
Draining Relationships	Any relationship based on illusions that each person has about the other, and involving inappropriate 'role playing', wastes a great deal of life energy and inhibits the full expression of who you are. Such relationships often involve a sense of being crushed or held back in life by the other person.	As you honour your core and listen to your inner imperatives you are more able to recognize any relationship that doesn't serve you, and adjust it to fit the real you or else spend less time with the person concerned.
Fear	'Freezes' you into inactivity and avoidance. Separates you from your core by forcing you to make compromising life choices. Inhibits the immune system, making you more susceptible to illness.	Identify your fears by writing them down. Decide which are valid and take action to allay them. Use the 'Give Away' exercise, on p.50, to help dispel any unnecessary fears.
Compromise	Continually sacrificing your own needs or desires in favour of what others want from you, or what you believe is required of you socially, inhibits your core energy.	Identify the signs of self compromise such as your use of the words 'I should' and 'I feel guilty if I don't'. Pause before you promise to do something you don't want to and think again.
Resentment	Feeling wronged by someone can lock you into a self-limiting energy-blocking prison.	Express your feelings of anger or pain directly to the person concerned. If this isn't practical or appropriate try the Forgiveness Letter and the Rewrite Your Past exercises (p.50) to help.
Depression	Suppresses metabolic processes, decreasing energy levels. Lowers self esteem. Results in the negative feedback loop (see p.45.)	Get started on an aerobic exercise programme. Examine your diet for food cravings and eliminate suspect food allergens (see Chapter 8 for more help).
Low Self-esteem	Lack of self-esteem encourages a defeatist/ victim attitude which drains energy. It also invites a lack of respect and appreciation from others around you.	Take a good look at the reasons you devalue yourself and ask if they are valid. Then write a list of your achievements and good qualities. Make a conscious effort to acknowledge these. Take action to enhance your self-esteem – try the Dressing Table Exercise (p.35) or begin an exercise programme (Chapter 10).
Unconscious Drainers	Any part of yourself which you don't want to face up to or integrate into your life ties up core energy. Look for any archetype, image or other person that you particularly hate, are afraid of or repelled by. Choose a name for the image.	Entertain the idea that your repelled image/ archetype is actually a neglected part of yourself that can bring you tremendous energy if you allow it to become a conscious part of you. Try dialoguing with an archetype.

The inner drainers

Even with the best will in the world to live from your core and the most conscientious attitude towards living a high-energy lifestyle, you may have no idea just how many factors can still drain your energy. Some, such as the way you eat or how much exercise you get are fairly self-evident. Others, such as the invisible electromagnetic fields that surround you, are more tricky to fathom. The most elusive of all are the silent attitudes and beliefs you hold within. These inner drainers can affect your energy at any moment of the day without your even being conscious of it. When they do, the smallest challenge or inconvenience becomes a tremendous burden, your stress levels soar and your energy levels plummet. Use the following exercise to help identify your inner energy-draining attitudes.

Self-check

How do you usually feel when you wake up in the morning?
☐ I just want to go back to sleep.
☐ I am excited about the day ahead.
Looking in the mirror, do you...
☐ Fret over wrinkles, grey hairs or blemishes and feel down?
☐ Feel pleased about yourself and good about the way you look – imperfections and all?
When faced with a difficult task at home or at work do you think...
☐ What a pain, perhaps if I avoid it someone else will do it?
☐ Here's a good challenge – a way to really stretch myself?
Looking forward to a romantic evening do you...
☐ Create a scenario of doom in case things work out badly?

☐ Enjoy imagining how wonderful the evening is going to be?
During an argument with your partner do you tell yourself...
☐ This is typical, he doesn't understand my needs. I'll never have a decent relationship?
☐ Maybe getting things out in the open can help us understand one another better and feel closer than before?
When you get a cold do you think...
☐ Just my luck! I always catch a cold at the worst possible moment?
☐ My body is obviously run down. Let me see how I can change my diet or my lifestyle in order to better support my needs?
When someone pays you a compliment do you...
☐ Dismiss it as untrue and then try to work out what their ulterior motive is?
☐ Accept the compliment graciously and thank them for their kindness?
What is your attitude to your job?
☐ I hate it. I'm overworked and underpaid, but I have to stick it – there's so much unemployment about I can't expect to find another.
☐ I enjoy my work. It gives me a chance to use my talents in a fulfilling way and I feel personally and financially rewarded.
You are tired and decide to spend a restful evening alone. A friend calls feeling down and asks you to go out with her. Do you...
☐ Go out with her even though you don't want to because you feel you should – this is the second time she has wanted to get together.
☐ Tell her you're tired, but would be happy to go out another night, and enjoy your evening alone.
You are invited to a family christening which you don't want to go to. Do you...

☐ Go because you're expected to. 'They make such a fuss if I don't.'
☐ Either excuse yourself because there is something else you want to do or go because you would enjoy making your family happy?
When you look back on your past do you...
☐ Feel resentful about the opportunities you didn't have and regret many of the things you have and haven't done?
☐ Feel grateful for the circumstances that have made you who you are and feel that if you could go back you wouldn't change a thing?
Do you feel your future happiness depends upon...
☐ Finding the right relationship, the right job, earning lots of money and hoping that not too many things go wrong?
☐ Continuing to live from your core and letting life unfold with optimistic anticipation?

If you identified mostly with the attitudes in the first answer to each question, it is likely that you suffer considerably from the Inner Energy-Drainers. Now make a note of your beliefs and assumptions in your journal with regard to some of the key issues in your life:
Your physical appearance. Do you believe that you can look the way you'd like to? If not, why not?
Your health. Do you believe that you can enjoy good health? If not, why not?
Your relationships. Do you believe you can have good relationships with your friends? Your family? Your lover? If not, why not?
Your home. Do you believe you can live in your ideal home? If not, why not?
Your work. Do you believe that you can have a satisfying, enjoyable

and well-paid job? If not, why not? **Your purpose.** Do you believe you have a purpose in life? If so, what is it? Do you believe you can fulfil it? If not, why not?

It is important to realize just how much the negative beliefs you hold about yourself and your life can limit not only the amount of energy you have, but also your potential for happiness and personal fulfilment. If you have skipped over the previous questions we advise you to go back and answer them in your journal. By becoming aware of any limiting belief you secretly carry inside you can begin the process of melting it away. Then your inner draining attitudes can become inner strengthening ones instead.

Emotional drainers

Just as it is common to hold negative beliefs, so many of us harbour negative feelings which deplete us of energy. A common one is anger. Anger in itself does not drain energy. It can be the driving force to achieving a goal. When anger is held in, however, it can turn into depression or resentment – both significant drainers. Another common energy drainer is fear or anxiety. Here are 3 techniques which we find useful for clearing negative emotional drainers. The first, The Forgiveness Letter, is especially good for anger or resentment. The second, Give Away, is good for dealing with fear and anxiety when they arise. The last one, Rewrite Your Past, helps you to reorientate the way you see yourself and your life in order to release any chronic negative feelings you may carry.

The forgiveness letter

Harboured negative feelings corrupt your perspective on life and lead you to attract negativity from others. They also make you feel bad about yourself. Getting rid of this energy-drainer means recognizing your negative feelings and choosing to let go of them

Write to any person towards whom you feel particularly resentful or angry (or even to 'life' itself). List all their offences. Don't hold back from telling the person exactly how you feel. At the bottom of the letter write: 'I (your name) hereby forgive you (the person's name) entirely for the above grievances. In so doing I bless you and wish you well, I release my ill feelings and honour my right to be whole, to be free and to trust in myself and my life.' When you have finished, read the letter out loud to yourself. Then burn it, letting the flames dissolve any remaining negative feelings.

Give away

Beginning to live from your core can be daunting. As you access deeper parts of your being it is not uncommon to experience feelings of fear or anxiety. Although it can be disconcerting to find yourself in a state of anxiety, once you recognize it you can use this simple technique to disperse your fearfulness. The Give-Away exercise is based on the American Indian tradition of offering gifts to Mother Earth. It can help you release negative emotional energy and gain comfort by reconnecting with the earth.

Stand or sit cross-legged on the floor. Notice your feelings of fear or anxiety and try to locate the area in your body where you experience them most strongly. Breathe into this place and each time you breathe out, imagine your feelings flowing down your body and into the ground beneath you. Make an offering of your fear to Mother Earth. As you do, you will feel calmer and more clear.

Rewrite your past

Feeling unhappy about your past can be a real block to living fully in the present or the future. When you feel hard done-by because of something that did or didn't happen to you, much of your energy gets tied up.

Just remember, your past belongs to you. Although the events may be fixed in your memory, how you feel towards those events can change. Let's say that you always had a dream to travel the world, but because you got married and began a family early your dream was sacrificed. Either you can feel sour about never doing what you wanted to or you can look at how much richness the pathway you did take has brought you.

Think of something in your past that makes you feel victimized. Write about your grievance as fully as possible in your journal, remembering the details as well as you can. When you have finished look at the grievance again. This time ask, 'Why did I choose this circumstance? What has it taught me? What strengths or qualities has it helped me develop?' Record your answers in your journal. See if you feel any different about your past (or your present and future) at the end.

Chapter 6

Lifting *the* veil *of* addiction

L ittle squanders core energy like addiction. And, although few women are aware of it, each of us has her own brand. Every kind – whether it be shooting heroin, munching chocolate chip cookies, or behaving like a workaholic – traps your energy within life-squandering negative feedback loops and limits your ability to make full use of your creativity.

At the centre of most addictive behaviour lies a feeling of guilt and powerlessness – both massive energy-drainers. Understanding addiction and becoming aware of where in your own life it may be operating is a vital part of taking stock. If you are addicted to something – whether it be sex, chocolate, tranquillizers or junk food – your ability to experience the full range of sensory delight in what you do, see, touch, smell and taste may be undermined. You can only fully appreciate the smouldering bitterness of the finest chocolate when you are *not* a chocoholic.

What is addiction?

Ask any doctor about addiction. He will tell you it involves a substance or a form of behaviour which is used compulsively, which alters behaviour and which causes unpleasant symptoms when access to it is denied. Alcohol, substance abuse, addictive eating behaviour, drugs and work-compulsion have been shown to lie beneath a wide range of chronic health problems and social ills. Sixty per cent of long-term patients in mental institutions in the West are there because of drug and alcohol problems and almost forty per cent of our hospital admissions are directly related to addiction. Addiction of one kind or another is our third greatest killer, after cancer and heart disease.

Banish the guilt

Most treatments for addiction go back to the nineteenth century and are riddled with Victorian morality. They are based on the notion that addictive problems are the result of voluntary *choice* on the part of the addict either because she is ethically inferior, has defective will power, or is one of society's outcasts. This moral judgement is particularly familiar to women who, caught in a trap of something as innocent as compulsive eating, continually harass themselves with accusations of being 'hopeless', 'weak-willed', 'inferior' and 'unloveable'. They sit down to a cup of tea and a biscuit only to find themselves devouring the whole packet.

In recent years, with the growing recognition of the compulsive nature of addictive behaviour, this self-righteous approach has given way to a psychiatric approach. It insists that although the addict is weak-willed, this is only the result of trauma or neurotic pressures from childhood, all of which can be talked through. More compassionate it may be, but with a few notable exceptions, it doesn't work. While an *understanding* of the psychological pressures behind your addictive behaviour (which are very real) may bring you a sense of comfort, it doesn't do much to cure the problem.

Then twenty or so years ago a handful of physicians, psychiatric workers and biochemists began to ask two interesting questions. First, is there such a thing as an 'addictive personality'? Second, if there is, does the source of addictive behaviour perhaps lie in a person's *physiology* – in a brain which behaves in a different way chemically from the norm in certain metabolic eccentricities, or in a blood chemistry which is out of the ordinary? As a result of such questions and thanks to the work of nutritionally aware psychiatrists, such as William Philpott MD, and clinical ecologists such as William Randolph MD, certain biochemical characteristics of the addict's body have come to light. So has a strong link between addiction and allergy.

The biochemistry of addiction

This appears to be particularly important in the case of alcoholism. The alcoholic who craves a drink appears in a very real way to be experiencing an *allergy* to alcohol or to the substances such as hops or grain or grapes from which it is made. So long as she continues to drink, the unpleasant effects of her allergy remain at bay. That is until the resources of her body have become exhausted at which point she experiences breakdown. If, however, she does not continue to feed her system the alcohol it craves (and to which she is allergic), she begins to experience allergic symptoms in the form of withdrawal – the shakes, fear, physical illness.

Out of these metabolic investigations into the physical characteristics of addiction has also come much understanding of how addictive behaviour works biochemically. Scientists such as Allan Luks, Executive Director of the Institute for the Advancement of Health in the United States, have shown, for instance that the appeal of stimulants such as cocaine, cigarettes and the amphetamines lies in their ability to rouse certain brain circuits in highly specific ways.

All of us, addicts and non-addicts, have *appetitive* brain systems involved in such activities as exploration, investigation of the environment, foraging and mating (which may be one of the reasons why both food and sex are high on the list of triggers for addictive behaviour). Under normal circumstances, these systems help your body re-establish balance after stressful experiences and events – be it childbirth, injury or intense fatigue – by releasing brain chemicals called *opioids*, like the endorphins and enkephalins. These signal the gratification of food when we are hungry, the pleasure of human warmth when we are lonely, the dissolution of pain when we are injured.

Artificial ecstasy

When our appetitive systems are animated artificially through sex, drugs, food, excitement or alcohol, the same brain receptors are stimulated. This can produce ecstatic feelings – sensations so pleasant and so relieving of stress that, when for any reason you find yourself in a situation of high pressure or real physical or psychic discomfort, you feel compelled to seek relief by artificially activating these circuits with whatever stimulants you have to hand. It is at this point that the normal appetitive functions of your brain circuits can surrender to compulsive drug-seeking behaviour as the feeling of distress stokes its own fires in an attempt to restore comfort, ease and a sense of wholeness.

Looking at addiction as a biochemical phenomenon has led to the development of methods of manipulating an addict's diet to her advantage. They involve the use of various natural substances, from free-form amino acids like glutamine to metabolites such as zinc, niacin and vitamin C. Herbs such as valerian, passiflora and skullcap are also used to correct metabolic imbalances caused by abuse and to lend the body an experience of comfort and wholeness during withdrawal. But what the biochemical approach has *not* been able to offer addicts is the ability to help people to cut off their addictive behaviour at its *roots*.

The role of consciousness

Biochemical treatments seldom take into account the most important factor of all: the role that *consciousness* plays both in the development and in the treatment of addiction. In Moscow, where drug and alcohol addiction has top research priority, Aaron Belkin and his colleagues at the Research Institute in Psychiatry have examined in depth the relationship between alcohol and the brain chemicals such as the endorphins, as well as the way they correlate with different states of consciousness and affect addictive behaviour. Like his colleagues in America, John Farquhar at Stanford University and psychiatrist Mohammed Shafii at the University of Michigan, Belkin recognizes that not only disturbed brain and body biochemistry trigger alterations in consciousness which leads to addictive behaviour, so do distorted states of consciousness – fear, uncertainty, low self-esteem and, most important of all, a sense of *meaningless* and *powerlessness*. All of these negative feelings drain energy. They make a person feel alienated from herself and her environment and trigger biochemical changes that can create a profound sense of physical and emotional discomfort, leading that person to take refuge in addiction. These researchers and clinicians are involved in fascinating and effective work with all kinds of addiction – from sex and food, to hard drugs, cigarettes and alcohol – using a wide variety of non-invasive techniques which help people make shifts in consciousness and in subtle energies. They include acupuncture, exercise therapy, meditation and even listening to tapes that balance brain activities.

Go for wholeness

What all of them insist is that any head-on approach to addiction by *fighting* it is all wrong. As American addiction therapist, David Hawkins, who is Director of the Institute for Spiritual Research in Sedona, Arizona, says: 'Attacking a drug problem directly only aggravates it because you are attacking a person's survival... you cannot attack the drug problem directly and expect to win.'

The new approach uses an enormous variety of techniques to induce a sense of profound wholeness and physical balance in the addict, in effect to bring her to the state she has been seeking through the substance or behaviour to which she is addicted. Farquhar, for instance, has created a step-by-step addiction programme using deep relaxation which rebalances the autonomic nervous system and helps link each participant with her own personal experience of meaning and nourishment on all levels – emotional, physical and spiritual. Shafii has had excellent long-term results with addicts using meditation.

In all cases therapists are calling on a wide range of natural methods and tools – from full-spectrum lights and carefully chosen sounds used to rebalance brain waves to deep meditation and body work – all in an effort to create a *complete* experiential environment for the addict with one end in mind: that she experiences the satisfaction of a balanced body chemistry and a sense of wholeness. For when the addict gets what she wants – an experience of ease, pleasure and completeness, and a sense that she is not a victim but has power over her own life, then she has no desire to disturb any of this by returning to drugs, alcohol or whatever else. As Belkin says, such modalities, coupled with explorations into the nature of personal meaning and an experience of personal power, work *physiologically* and *psychologically* to alter addictive behaviour permanently because 'the necessary hormones are released in the necessary places, normalizing biological processes in the human organism.'

The new work in addiction is helping addicts transform the driving energy behind their addictions into creative energy. It can also bring to the rest of us, with our minor compulsions, a much greater understanding that addiction is not the province of the weak-willed or the emotional or biochemical misfit as we have been led to believe.

A universal phenomenon

In many ways the whole phenomenon of addiction is a metaphor for the greater sickness of meaninglessness and powerlessness which pervades our whole society. As Andrew Weil, Professor of Addiction Studies at University of Arizona, says, 'Addiction is a fundamental aspect of being human.' It does not begin in self-indulgence or weakness as we have been led to believe. It begins in a distorted attempt to find meaning, fulfilment, and a more satisfying physical and mental state. 'All addicts are striving to experience wholeness,' says Weil. 'And to a greater or lesser extent urbanized man and woman, addict or no, lacks a sense of personal wholeness and universal connection.' As Weil likes to point out, the lack of a fully realized perception of personal power and meaning is destructive to anyone. That is how we have all become addicts of some sort. The difference between a heroin addict and a television addict is that the person who sits in front of the television to wind down after work is channelling only a moderate amount of her energy into the addiction, whereas the heroin addict's entire life energy may be going down the drain in search of the next fix.

Becoming aware of any addictions in your own life, whether they be to sugar, cigarettes, chocolate, a relationship, work, alcohol or sex, is the first step to re-claiming energy which is being wasted on them and being able to re-channel it creatively. When you start to look upon an addiction in this way, as a storeroom for your own power and energy just waiting to be accessed, then overcoming an addiction, major or mi-nor, becomes an exciting challenge. Of course it isn't easy. Denying yourself something which your body has come to depend on is never fun. But, with the right approach, you can transform the symptoms of with-drawal into steps that lead you towards a sense of satis-faction in your own life.

Chapter 6
Workbook

Workbook *for* Lifting *the* veil *of* addiction

At the root of the word addiction is the latin verb *addicere*, one definition of which is 'to surrender.' When we surrender to anything other than the life force at the core of our being, or God if you like, we do ourselves a great injustice. Not only is the object of our surrender – the television set, chocolate chip icecream, a few gin and tonics – unworthy of our devotion, it is also incapable of providing us with the satisfaction and support we need.

Any attempt to overcome an addiction starts with the realization that an addiction is not simply a bad habit adopted by the weak-willed or self-indulgent individual looking for a way out. Rather it is a legitimate (and often unconscious) search for a sense of wholeness. Although an addiction can never satisfy the need for wholeness, it can at least alert us to the longing and set us on the path towards finding it. Each step we take can release trapped energy.

Depending upon the severity of an addiction, the road to recovery may be relatively painless (choosing to watch less television) or life threateningly severe, as in the case of a detox-clinic programme for a severe drug addiction. Here, we are interested in the more moderate (and often unrecognized) addictions which are within the individual's power to overcome without necessarily requiring medical assistance.

The eight-step plan
Step one: Identify
Look at the definition of addiction that follows and apply to it any of the following substances or behaviours you think you might be addicted to – even mildly:

The dependence on a substance or form of behaviour which is used compulsively and produces a feeling of satisfaction and/or a psychic drive. When access is denied to the addictive element, cravings and unpleasant physical and/or psychological symptoms of withdrawal occur.

Possible addictive substances
Sugar, chocolate, icecream, biscuits (any other sweets or any other food), coffee, alcohol, cigarettes, mild narcotics such as marijuana, tranquillizers

Possible addictive behaviour
Working, shopping, sex, falling in love, watching television, eating.

Step two: Acknowledge
Once you have determined a suspect addiction from the list above, or found any other element that fits the addiction description for you, use the questions below to determine the severity of your addiction. How much of your energy – both mental and physical – goes into feeding the addiction?

The questions are formulated around the term 'crutch' which represents an addictive substance or addictive form of behaviour.

Answer each of the following questions A, B or C: A Almost always, B Sometimes, C Never

☐ Do you suffer from low self-esteem and feel unable to cope with many of the pressures of life?

☐ When you are challenged by a stressful situation do you automatically turn to the crutch?

☐ Do you find yourself thinking about when you will next be able to have your crutch in the day?

□ Do you get nervous or anxious at the thought of being deprived of your crutch?

□ When you use the crutch does it bring you a sense of comfort almost immediately?

□ Do you find it difficult to stop taking it/doing it once you start?

□ Do you find yourself feeling guilty about it?

□ Are you defensive when anyone seems to criticize your use of it?

□ When you feel lonely, depressed, anxious or upset, do you automatically reach for the crutch?

□ Do you suffer withdrawal symptoms such as depression, irritability or headaches when you don't have the crutch for a few hours/a few days?

If you answered mostly C to the above questions then addiction probably inhibits your life energy very little – lucky you!

If you answered mostly B, then your addiction is moderate. Your energy levels could be increased to some extent by cutting down on or eliminating your crutch.

If you answered mostly A, then your addiction is significant and your energy considerably drained by it. You could benefit greatly from overcoming it and eliminating the crutch (or the compulsive use of it) from your life.

Step three: Reclaim

Are you ready to give it up?
This is a legitimate dilemma. The question can help you to see how important the energy lost through the addiction is to you. There are only two answers – yes or no. Saying, 'Well I would, but I don't have the willpower' is as good as saying 'It's not really that impor-

tant – perhaps I'll try another time.' If that is truly how you feel, then feel free to skip the rest of this chapter and go on to the next one. For unless you are prepared to put yourself wholeheartedly behind overcoming an addiction, unless the rewards of more energy, greater self esteem and a sense of being in control of your life tempt you more than the chocolate bars or the cigarettes, you will never do it.

If in response to the question you say, 'I want to, but I'm scared' the light is green and you will find the support you need to overcome your fear and your addiction.

Step four: Root out

The process of overcoming an addiction involves some honest soul-searching to discover what is behind it. An addiction may mask any number of uncomfortable feelings. Getting to the root of it may come only gradually. Try to remember back to when the addiction began. Ask yourself what particular stresses you were having to deal with at the time. What was the need you might have had that wasn't being fulfilled? Were you resentful or angry towards someone or something? Did you feel lonely? or empty? or lost? Make a note of your findings in your journal. If you cannot identify any particular feelings, don't worry. It may be that they are well hidden and will only surface as you begin to eliminate your crutch. Be sure to make the connection when they do and to record in your journal any feelings, thoughts or memories that arise. (Negative feelings, such as resentment, can be a real stumbling block to giving up your addiction. Try The Forgiveness Letter on p.50).

Step five: Help yourself

Your sugar intake can be responsible for increasing your cravings for anything from cigarettes, to shopping, to love. The group of glands that control the body's blood sugar levels and carbohydrate metabolism are also involved in the control of appetite and other urges or hungers. When this group of glands – the hypothalamic-pituitary-adrenal (or H-P-A) axis – is challenged by the intake of too much sugar, it becomes unable to establish a sense of harmony or wellbeing in the body. As a result, a person can experience discomfort and look to their addictive crutch for help. The link between sugar and addiction is also seen in the way that an alcoholic or cigarette addict, after deciding to give up drinking or smoking, may develop a new addiction to foods containing sugar and so gain weight.

Here are some simple steps to help balance the body's blood-sugar levels and eliminate cravings. (If sugar or chocolate or caffeine drinks are your addictions – bear with the irony of the first suggestion!)

A happy H-P-A Avoid all forms of sugar and refined carbohydrates as well as chocolate and caffeine-containing drinks, all of which stress the H-P-A axis.

Acid zappers Go for alkaline-forming foods such as fresh, raw vegetables, fruits and, in particular, sprouted pulses, seeds and grains. These foods neutralize the build up of acid wastes which can be responsible for cravings.

Amino aid The amino acid L-glutamine, taken in doses of 2-4 grams a day, has been shown to reduce sugar (and alcohol) cravings in ninety per cent of people tested. As with all free-form amino acids, it should be taken on an empty stomach well before or after meals.

Sunflower snack If you have a tendency towards hypoglycaemia (if in doubt try the quiz on p.63), have a protein snack every few hours – try a few fresh unsalted nuts or seeds for example. Sunflower seeds are particularly helpful for a cigarette addiction as they contain ingredients which mimic some of nicotine's effect (such as stimulating the adrenal function and brain activity), and so satisfy the body's craving.

Try the fizz trick This amazing elimination aid for withdrawal symptoms, general fatigue or hangovers was taught to us by Shona Williams, a director of The Open Forum in New Zealand. Place half a teaspoon each of citric acid powder and bicarbonate of soda in a glass of water or fruit juice. Let the mixture fizz and then drink it. Although the taste isn't wonderful, the effect is!

Tonic C Use a vitamin C tonic whenever you feel a craving.

Like the Fizz Trick, Vitamin C helps eliminate wastes from the body and alleviate withdrawal symptoms.

Step six: Have fun

Denial is a drag. If you are going to give something up you need to find something else to replace it with so that you don't feel cheated. Instead of focusing on what you're missing out on, find new things to bring you pleasure.

● Take up a creative hobby such as painting, sculpting, playing a musical instrument, writing, dress-making, singing.

● Find a form of exercise that brings you pleasure (see Chapter 10 Energy In Motion). Exercise is ideal for overcoming an addiction because it helps mobilize and eliminate the body toxins which can provoke depression and cravings. It also heightens self-esteem.

● Assuming shopping isn't your addiction, buy yourself something that you have always wanted.

● Treat yourself to the luxury of a weekend away in the country.

● Take a trip to the beauty salon for a massage or facial.

● Find time to relax and enjoy doing nothing at all. A deep relaxation exercise or guided imagery journey (see p.124) can be helpful to let go of the withdrawal symptoms of anxiety or nervousness.

Step seven: Elicit support

Overcoming an addiction is hard. Without support it can even be impossible. Establish a good support system around you and don't be afraid to ask for help.

● Spend time with people who aren't themselves addicted to what you're giving up. If your addiction is alcohol, avoid the company of alcoholics and make your life easier by not socializing in pubs.

● Clean out your house – get rid of all the addictive substances, sugary foods, chocolate, caffeine drinks or whatever NOW – don't wait to finish that last packet of cigarettes.

● Find a help group. The 'Anonymous' groups can be really inspiring and provide the courage and support needed.

● Make sure your friends and family understand the step you are taking and support you. If any friends are unsupportive, spend less time with them.

Step eight: Feel proud

See the journey to overcome your addiction and reclaim your lost energy as a heroic one. Beware of the pitfalls and take steps to avoid them, but don't chastise yourself when you slip up. Use your journal to record your difficulties as well as your triumphs. Adopt the AA principal of 'One day at a time' and celebrate your progress bit by bit.

B BOOSTERS FOR CRAVINGS

The B-Complex vitamins are particularly important for sugar metabolism, and hence for satisfying cravings, as are the minerals chromium, zinc, magnesium and manganese. Consider taking a multi-vitamin and mineral supplement (see Resources, p.137).

Niacin, one of the B vitamins, together with vitamin B-6 and the amino acid tyrosine, has been shown to reduce cravings for both alcohol and nicotine. Most authorities recommend daily doses of 250-500mg of niacin with 25-50mg of B6 and 500-1000mg of tyrosine. (They point out that taking niacin can result in a temporary 'niacin flush' as it dilates the capillaries.)

Have a spoonful of unsulphured black strap molasses. Not only is molasses rich in B vitamins, as well as the minerals iron, potassium, calcium and magnesium, but it is also alkaline-forming. It can help rebalance the minerals in your body while satisfying a sweet tooth.

Mapping *the* minefield *of* nutrition

These days it is hard for anyone to eat well. The media is full of contradictory advice: Eat more carrots… don't eat butter… drink milk… stay away from mucus-forming milk products… eat eggs… eggs? You must be joking, eggs contain that dangerous stuff cholesterol don't they? …and so on. Making sense of it all is like trying to make your way through a minefield.

Since the Industrial Revolution, when roller mill-ing gave us the ability to fractionate wheat – to separate the starch from the bran and germ and therefore to produce refined flour and white bread – manufacturers have been messing with our foods. Throughout evolution our ancestors have eaten these foods in their natural form. We are therefore genetically accustomed to eating them that way.

The foods that now fill our supermarket shelves bear little resemblance to our ancestors' fodder. They are fractionated, refined and modified beyond all recognition. Such messing about leads to the development of widespread degenerative diseases, in which the twenti-eth-century diet of phoney foods has now been strongly implicated. They range from diabetes to varicose veins, and from cancer to arthritis or coronary heart disease, not to mention a wide variety of mental troubles includ-ing schizophrenia, chronic depression and anxiety.

Chemical additives, food colourings and flavour-ings, hydrogenated 'junk fats' – they are all products of a multi-billion pound food industry whose main purpose is not to serve your health but to fill its own coffers at your expense.

As an experiment, a biochemist at the University of Georgia bought one of the new munchy-crunchy chil-dren's cereals. He emulsified both the box and the cereal, then fed one white rat the box and another the cereal. The one that ate the box thrived. The other one did not. So poor is the quality of common convenience foods that the junk packaging can be nutritionally superior to the food it contains.

Food for nought

The multi-national food industry claims to spend a lot of money on nutritional research and development. Don't be deceived. Ninety-two per cent of its 'research and development' costs go to develop quick-preparation foods and consumer appeal – what the US National Science Foundation calls 'motivational research and product promotion'. (These days some fast-food chains even add aluminium – a heavy metal which can seriously disturb human brain function – to the processed cheese they use on cheeseburgers just so it will melt better.)

Like the multi-national drug industry our food industry is either directly or indirectly responsible for most of what you read in the media about food and health. It supplies ready-made diets, articles and information for journalists for use in preparing magazine, newspaper and television coverage. It prints up pretty little booklets on slimming, or how to protect your husband's heart, for wide distribution. Some of this information is better than others but all is designed first and foremost to further its own financial interests.

What price convenience?

One of the spin-offs of fractionating foods has been a kind of 'fractionated' thinking about nutrition which has led to rampant confusion. Much of the talk these days is not about food – the stuff you eat for pleasure and wellbeing – but about *parts* of food: cholesterol, saturated or unsaturated fats, carbohydrates, vitamins and minerals, or about how to make a meal faster and easier. In Chapter 9, Energy Grazing, we take everything back to basics and look at *real* food for *real* health and at what kind of eating can best support endless energy. Let's now look at some of the perils of eating convenience foods and examine some of the specific pitfalls you may personally encounter. They include Candida albicans, the intestinal yeast-fungus which lowers immunity, food allergies, which can cause emotional aberrations and excess weight, and low blood sugar, which can have you crunching chocolate bars and slurping instant coffee just to keep going, not to mention causing bad skin, flabby flesh and poor quality nails and hair.

The pre-mixed, pre-washed, pre-cooked (almost pre-eaten) food we buy is very expensive. Take the humble potato. We rang the local supermarket this morning to find that boiling potatoes, sold as they come out of the ground, are currently selling at 18 pence a kilo – enough to make mashed potato for around four to six people. A packet of dehydrated and powdered pre-packaged potato to serve the same number will set you back 52 pence – almost three times as much. And you can take things even further. The same weight of potato crisps, can cost an astounding £9.75 – fifty times as much. Furthermore, you can run the same exercise

for just about every food you can think of and come up with more or less the same results.

Food manufacturers take inexpensive low-profit staples and turn them into expensive high-profit quasi-foods. The truth is, the more *processed* a food is the more *costly* it is, not only to your purse but also to your health. For the more processed it is, the further it has come from its whole state and the more it has lost of the remarkable synergistic balance of nutrients with which nature endowed it.

By now everybody knows that convenience foods are replete with chemical flavour enhancers, colourants, and preservatives such as BHA and BHT. When these artificial additives, to which our bodies have never become accustomed throughout the whole of human evolution, are eaten over and over for months and years they can not only disturb your metabolic processes, they can also lead to the kind of biochemical chaos that creates mental and emotional confusion. This is something easily seen in young people who have been raised on junk foods. In fact there have been some interesting studies done recently which show that the behaviour of juvenile delinquents raised on junk food can be dramatically improved by taking them off it.

Go for synergy

Other nasty things can happen which undermine your health when you eat foods whose wholeness has been destroyed. For good nutrition is not about how much of this or that vitamin you should take or how many grams of protein you need. It is about eating delicious foods grown on healthy soils as close as possible to their whole state. Of course, throw away the peel of the banana and take out the fish intestines before you cook your salmon, but as a general rule this wholeness principle works. It asks that you eat the skin of the potato as well as the flesh, and the germ and bran of the wheat grain from which you make your bread as well as the starch. When you fractionate a food you destroy its synergy: the way in which the vitamins, minerals, essential fatty acids, carbohydrates, fibre, amino acids and all the – as yet unidentified – plant factors which help build health have been bound together by nature to support each other. Within such wholeness is to be found a quantum power for health. Destroy it and you undermine your own potential for energy, good looks and youthful vitality.

Sugar blues

When convenience foods are manufactured, two important highly processed ingredients are added to them in vast quantities: fat and sugar. They are cheap for food manufacturers to use. Also, eating foods full of them tends to make us crave them even more, all of which is great for profits. (In the average supermarket it is even hard to find a loaf of *whole grain* bread to which sugar has not been added, not to mention the vast quantities that go into its pale white counterpart.) Each of us in Britain on average consumes over 200 pounds of sugar a year – sugar which has been surreptitiously tucked into the foods we buy.

Everybody knows that eating lots of white sugar causes dental carries. It also contributes to obesity, diabetes and hypoglycaemia (low blood sugar), as well as a lot of even more deadly illnesses such as coronary heart disease. What few are aware of, however, is that in recent years sugar has become increasingly implicated in emotional disorders as well – from anxiety and depression to hyperactivity in children, psychotic episodes and schizophrenia. Sugar affects the behaviour of many people. Eating lots of it over the years can deplete your body of essential nutrients, like chromium, which are necessary for the maintenance of mental and emotional balance, and for stabilizing blood sugar levels which helps protect you from fatigue and depression.

Beware junk fats

The perils of fat-stuffed convenience foods (from biscuits and quiches to frozen meals) are less well known but equally bad news. Just as food producers have fractionated our wheat to produce cheap white flour, they have also broken up and chemically distorted the oils and fats which occur naturally in our foods and turned them into junk fats.

The role of fat in creating good health is an area of enormous confusion. Here are the facts. Your body can make all the fat it needs for daily metabolic processes except for certain essential polyunsaturated fatty acids (PUFAs). These are found naturally in fresh food such as seeds and nuts, vegetables and fish – even in wild meat such as game. For optimal health you probably need no more than 2-4 tablespoons of PUFAs a day. Yet they can be as hard to find in a modern diet of convenience foods as the proverbial hen's teeth.

PUFAs are important for your brain and nerve cells, your skin and hair. They are also necessary as building blocks for cell membranes all over your body. They are precursors of important and highly reactive local hormones called prostaglandins which you need to make many of your metabolic processes work. The trouble with PUFAs is that they are very chemically reactive. This means they turn rancid in contact with air, light or heat, for they oxidize rapidly, although often their rancidity is not noticeable by taste or smell.

In their natural state in plant and animal foods, PUFAs come packaged together in synergy with vitamin E and other natural anti-oxidants that help prevent them from spoiling. Processing of these foods to produce refined vegetable oils removes this protection. Through complex processes which often involve the use of unpleasant chemical solvents, it also creates the highly artificial products which you find in see-through plastic bottles stacked on supermarket shelves. Not only are these oils, fats and margarines of little benefit to your health, but they also can be *highly* detrimental to it.

Margarine madness

A word about margarines which claim they are 'high in polyunsaturates'. No PUFA is solid at room temperature. When margarine is manufactured, the vegetable oils it is made from are changed chemically from *unsaturated* fats to *saturated* ones by the addition of extra hydrogen atoms. The ordinary saturated fat that you find in steak or chicken is far healthier than the artificially produced *trans*-unsaturated fatty acids found in margarines.

Read labels when you shop. Anything that says it contains hydrogenated vegetable oil or partially hydrogenated vegetable oil, leave on the shelf. You don't want chemical residues from any of these artificially produced oils in your body. Natural fresh farm butter is far healthier than margarine. A diet high in *trans* junk fats, and therefore deficient in PUFAs, drains energy, encourages you to gain weight and can make you susceptible to early ageing as well as encouraging dry skin, poor hair and weak nails. Beware.

Food cravings and other miseries

Feed rats on human convenience foods and they want more. Those who have inherited a tendency to lay down fat cells also become obese. Try it yourself. Live on a diet of junk foods – chips and hamburgers, white bread and chocolate bars – for a week and you will find yourself feeling dissatisfied after every meal. If you are a woman with unlucky genes, you will also gain weight. If not you will simply pollute your body. Should you continue eating in this way for months or even years, you render yourself prone to illness, early ageing and degenerative disease. Eating processed foods leads to food cravings which your body mistakenly registers as hunger.

The 'eat one biscuit – eat the packet' scenario is a familiar one. Such biscuit-woofing creates feelings of guilt and inadequacy as well as fear about weight gain in women. It is also very hard to overcome. That is unless you know what is really going on. In truth your digestive system in its infinite wisdom (did you realize that the human gut contains more nerve endings than any other part of the body?) is responding to the nutritionally corrupt foods you are putting into it with irritation and sensitivity. Yet, instead of your recognizing the signals for what they are – namely a sign to change your way of eating to banish this discomfort – you think you feel hungry and so you eat more in an attempt to settle the disturbance.

Food sensitivities

Sometimes called food intolerance or even food allergies, these sensitivities can be enormous pitfalls in the nutrition minefield. Navigating round them takes a real understanding of how they work and an awareness of how they may be operating in your own life. Food sensitivities or food allergies are quite different from ordinary allergies which occur when a woman has an antibody response to the substance with which she has come in contact. They are a negative reaction your body makes to something you eat. In a food allergy or intolerance, unlike ordinary allergies, the antibody-antigen response cannot always be demonstrated by current immunological or laboratory methods. Such sensitivity reactions usually occur because you do not have the enzymes you need to digest a certain food, because your total stress load is simply too high, because your digestive system is confused and sensitized from additives or contaminants in the foods you eat, or for many other reasons, some of which are as yet unknown.

Sister to addiction

Food and chemical allergies or sensitivities are enormously widespread – and becoming more so all the time as our environment becomes increasingly filled with chemicals and artificial foods for which the cells of the human body have a natural aversion. The curious thing about food and chemical sensitivities is that whatever you happen to be allergic to, whether it be wheat or alcohol or chocolate, you will find you have a *craving* for it – an *addiction* to it.

This discovery came out of some fascinating work done by clinical ecologists and nutritionally orientated psychiatrists. In the past thirty years they have demonstrated that many of our physical and emotional illnesses are in fact sensitivity reactions. Working with thousands of patients, presenting them with an enormous variety of symptoms, they have developed a profound understanding of this kind of allergy-cum-addiction, or what are called maladaptive allergic reactions. This is how it works. When you are allergic to a food or chemical, on first contact, you will react negatively to it. If you use it or are exposed to it continually, however, these first negative symptoms become 'masked' so you no longer experience them. Instead, you develop a craving or addiction for the substance. So long as you continue to expose yourself to it you can avoid the unpleasant allergic response you had first time round. This is such a strange and unexpected phenomenon that most people are

---

FOOD – SENSITIVITY SYMPTOMS

Physical symptoms: upset stomach, wind, heartburn, underweight, overweight or quick shifts in body weight, excessive hunger, frequent colds, runny nose, sinusitis, dark circles under the eyes, leg aches, muscle pains, food cravings, low blood sugar, Crohn's disease, coughing, breathing difficulties, hot flushes, headaches, nervousness, constipation, diarrhoea, colitis, blurred or double vision, PMT, swollen legs or fingers, itchy eyes.

Emotional and mental symptoms: irritability, hyperactivity, fatigue, listlessness, weakness, sluggishness, desire to sleep all the time, lack of coordination, hypersensitivity to noise, hot and cold or odours, depression, mood swings, confusion, inability to concentrate, anxiety, poor memory, addiction to alcohol or drugs, compulsive eating or other compulsive behaviour.

not even conscious they may be suffering from a sensitivity. Frequently, this kind of allergy-cum-addiction is the hidden cause behind the unpleasant 'eat one biscuit, eat the packet' syndrome. Wheat is one of the most common foods to which people are allergic.

The same can be true of substances we inhale. Take tobacco. Seventy-five per cent of all people are allergic to tobacco. The first contact they have with it brings on the symptoms of biliousness, dizziness or coughing. If they go on smoking, these symptoms are suppressed by the continual contact. So long as they keep smoking they will be relatively free of them until such time as their adrenals and basic immunity become overwhelmed by the stress of it all.

Instant turn off

This temporary respite from negative symptoms by continual exposure to the substance is a perfect example of how the *maladaptive allergic state* works. Only when a person decides to stop smoking does an acute reaction occur. Then she goes cold turkey and has to face the full flood of negative symptoms which have been masked. The most surprising aspect of all is the way in which nasty withdrawal symptoms can, with startling immediacy, be suppressed again simply by reintroducing the tobacco (or the wheat, or caffeine, or alcohol, or what have you) into a person's body. We have watched clinical ecologists in hospitals do this, in stunned amazement.

Clinical ecologists identify food and environmental sensitivities by putting a patient on an elimination diet which excludes the most common allergens such as wheat, milk, sugar and food chemicals for five days. Then they introduce small quantities of these foods, often in microscopic dilution, a few drops under the tongue, and monitor changes in blood pressure, pulse and behaviour that take place as well as the subjective experience of the person being tested. Once an offending food or chemical has been identified, the person is advised either to eliminate it from her diet (if the allergy-addiction is serious) or to make sure that she does not eat or drink the offending food or expose herself to the offending substance more often than once every four or five days.

In the case of minor food intolerance (which is what most of us are dealing with) only eating the suspect foods *infrequently* works well. It eliminates cravings and other allergic symptoms by removing the constant challenge and overload the problem substance presents your system. In the case of serious food and chemical sensitivities, however, you often need skilled medical help to eliminate the offenders from your life completely.

Should you be unlucky enough to suffer any of the symptoms listed above, it can be worthwhile putting yourself on an elimination diet for a few days to see if they disappear and then gradually introduce the foods to which you suspect you may have a sensitivity. (The most obvious ones are the ones you eat most frequently and those for which you have a particular craving.)

Identifying pitfalls and dangers

Food sensitivity is only one of the many perils concealed within the nutrition minefield. Others include cravings for fatty foods which can indicate a fatty-acid deficiency, crash dieting, low blood sugar and a proliferation of yeast in the gut. Environmental pollution, because of its effect on your nutrient requirements and the way chemicals and heavy metals in the environment can undermine the enzyme activity needed for healthy metabolic processes, is also a danger. It is worth taking a moment to look at some of the things that might be operating in your own life. Many of them are overlapping in the sense that if you have food allergies you are also likely to be susceptible to an over growth of the intestinal yeast-fungus Candida albicans. Happily, many of the changes you can make in your diet and lifestyle to eliminate one, also help get rid of another. All of the nutritional actions you take to encourage endless energy are not only a way of helping overcome some difficulty, they also strengthen your whole organism, forming the foundation of health and good looks at the highest possible level.

Chapter 7
Workbook

Workbook *for* Mapping *the* minefield *of* nutrition

Now let's home in on some of the specific barriers to endless energy. An awareness of which apply to you can help you to take the simple steps necessary to eliminate them. In fact awareness is half the battle. Go through the 6 quizzes below, answering each question yes or no, to give you an idea of what area you may want to work on. You will find help after each quiz or be referred to other parts of the book. Once you have completed the quizzes, record in your journal any area in your own nutritional life that could benefit from change. Make a decision to begin to work on 1 or 2 things and record your commitment. Go back through your journal each week to remind yourself of the commitments you have made and make a note of your progress. All of us need reminding again and again. It is part of being human.

Quiz one

☐ Do you wake up tired?
☐ Do you rely on a cup of coffee to get yourself started first thing in the morning?
☐ Do you crave sweet foods?
☐ Do you get irritable, feel faint or get a headache if you skip a meal or don't eat for several hours?
☐ Do you sometimes suffer from blurred vision?
☐ Do you tend to feel drowsy after meals?
☐ Do you get tired in the late morning or late afternoon?
☐ Do you get anxiety attacks or feel depressed sometimes for no reason?
☐ Do you have difficulty making decisions?
☐ Do you cry easily?

If you answered yes to 5 or more of these questions you may need to support your blood sugar to keep it stable. Read on.

Simple disasters

Simple carbohydrates – white sugar, white flour – are inimical to optimum human health. Eat lots of them over a long period of time (which is exactly what we do in the Western world) and you can end up with degenerative diseases even if you have never touched a food additive or come in contact with an environmental chemical.

Eating a lot of sugar, white flour or foods containing them stimulates the pancreas to produce insulin which your body needs to metabolize these simple carbohydrates. The more simple carbohydrates that pass your lips, the more insulin your pancreas needs to produce to stabilize blood-sugar levels, until eventually it loses its ability to respond to the demand and exhaustion (or even diabetes) results. Eating lots of sugar and white flour can also lead to a condition called functional hypoglycaemia. Here, your body, depleted of essential nutrients like chromium which are needed to support the enzymes involved, can no longer metabolize them and the pancreas becomes trigger-happy, creating repetitive abnormally low levels of glucose (sugar) in your blood. It is a form of chronic low blood sugar where you get a feeling of dizziness or fatigue, confusion or restlessness, which pushes you to reach for coffee and sweet or starchy things just to keep going. Low blood sugar is frequently the culprit behind the energy swings that women experience during the day, especially around the time of their menstrual period. It can also be responsible for wakefulness at night, night sweats, swollen legs and feet, constant hunger and emotional instability. This kind of low blood sugar is common among women who put feeding themselves properly at the bottom of their list of priorities, beneath caring for others, and work.

Low blood sugar

Eliminating chronic low blood sugar is a matter of re-educating your pancreas to work properly and cutting all simple carbohydrates out of your diet. This means nix on sugar, white flour and *everything* made with them. It also means making sure you eat a little food containing good protein every 2 or 3 hours to help stabilize blood sugar swings that cause symptoms. Most experts in functional hypoglycaemia insist that you take 300-400mcg of the mineral chromium as a supplement each day, too. Here are some of the dietary changes they recommend.

Go for fibre

This does not mean adding the ubiquitous wheat bran to everything you eat, since wheat bran (naively often recommended to increase fibre in the diet) can cause mild to severe intestinal upset for many people and even make constipation *worse* in some. It means eating wholefoods such as whole grain breads, brown rice, porridge oats, salads and fruit which contain natural fibre. Unlike wheat bran, the fibre in oat-bran porridge (which is delicious), as

well as certain fibre supplements can all help slow down hypoglycaemic reactions, particularly for someone who is getting plenty of protein in her diet. Spirulina can also help stabilize blood sugar reactions – 3 or 4 tablets of it before meals or a teaspoon to a tablespoon mixed into a large cup of vegetable broth as a snack (see p.79).

Don't go hungry

Never let yourself be caught without food. Eat 6 to 8 small 'meals' a day – every 2 to 3 hours. This is not as hard as it sounds if you carry about with you a handful of mixed sunflower, sesame and pumpkin seeds, or almonds, and munch them every few hours. You can even carry in your bag a small piece of chicken or a hard-boiled egg with a sprinkling of sea salt, for mid-morning and mid-afternoon snacks while everybody else is munching a biscuit. If you awaken in the night, eat half a banana or a whole-grain oatcake without sugar. It can be useful to have a snack like this before bedtime to improve sleep.

Food sensitivities

Many people with low blood sugar are actually allergic or sensitive to certain foods or chemicals in their environment which can trigger low blood-sugar fatigue and symptoms. Investigate this possibility.

Cast out the junk

Throw out of your larder sugar, refined and processed foods like instant mashed potatoes and instant rice, white flour, spaghetti

gravies, baked beans, alcohol, colas and squashes (including low calorie ones). Avoid fruit juices and stay away from very sweet fruit such as figs and dates, or any dried fruits, until the problem has cleared itself up.

Good proteins and carbos

High-protein foods such as fish and eggs, cottage cheese, tofu, seeds, nuts and yogurt are important. They take a long time to digest fully and help stabilize blood-sugar swings. So are complex carbohydrates such as brown rice, whole-grain 100 per cent pure rye breads and crisp breads, Jerusalem artichokes and baked potatoes eaten with their skins. Eat them often. If you are a meat eater try to include lamb's liver in your meals at least once and preferably twice a week. Liver is a superb source of B-Complex vitamins. Supplement your diet with chromium.

Quiz two

☐ Do you frequently get indigestion?

☐ Do you often have a runny nose or do you notice your sinuses become blocked after eating?

☐ Do you suffer from one or more of the following: migraine or sinus headaches, persistent acne, particularly around the mouth or chin, asthma or shortness of breath?

☐ Do you tend to put on weight even when you don't overeat?

☐ Do you sometimes feel worse after eating?

☐ Do you feel 'fuzzy headed' or depressed within 2 hours of eating a regular-sized meal?

□ Do you feel better if you skip meals or fast?

□ Are you a picky eater? Do you have a strong aversion to particular foods?

□ Is there any specific food that you find it hard to go without?

□ Do you ever start a packet of biscuits and have to finish them all?

If you answered yes to 5 or more of these questions re-read the section on food sensitivities and check your symptoms against the list on p.61. It might be worthwhile putting yourself on an elimination diet for 5 days to see if the symptoms disappear and then gradually reintroduce the particular foods to which you suspect you have a sensitivity.

Five day detox

Begin this elimination diet on a Friday so you can have a bit of a rest over the weekend should you find that you need it.

Day one

Nothing special demanded here except that you stop taking stimulants such as chocolate, anything containing sugar, coffee and tea and depressants such as alcohol. Don't eat bread, or pasta or grain-based foods such as breakfast cereals and biscuits during the day. For your last meal of the day have a large raw salad of fresh vegetables (see p.92 for suggestions).

Days two and three

These days you eat only fruit, as much as you like but only one kind each day. If you are easily bored, change the kind of fruit you eat once during a day, by choosing one kind in the morning and another kind in the afternoon, as long as you leave a 2-hour gap between the two. Choose from the following fruits: apples, watermelon or other melon, pears. Avoid bananas, strawberries, oranges, tangerines and grapefruit.

Days four and five

These days are simple. You eat only fruits for breakfast – apples, melon, pears (you can mix them together if you like in a fruit salad or put them in a blender to make a frappé). For lunch you have a large salad made from raw vegetables topped with olive oil and lemon juice or cider vinegar. Then for dinner you have steamed or wok-fried vegetables cooked in a little olive oil (see recipe, p.95).

Day six onwards

Eat as on days 4 and 5 but at each meal introduce a different 'suspected' food. For instance at breakfast, in addition to your fruit, you might eat a piece of dry wheat toast – then see how you feel. At lunch try a piece of cheese or an orange or a hunk of chocolate. Then make a note in your journal of any reactions to the food added. Test only one food at a time. Try these first: wheat, sugar, chocolate, coffee, eggs, cheese, milk, yogurt, or any other food which in the past you have had a craving for and have tended to eat more than 4 times a week.

If you have a sensitivity problem you will find that your pulse rate will go up within 3 minutes of eating the food (see p.104 for how to take your pulse) and/or you will develop some kind of mild (or not so mild) symptoms. These could be mental or physical (as in the list on p.61). Then, after having tested the most obvious suspects, in the next couple of days gradually introduce back into your life the rest of the foods you ordinarily eat, omitting as much as possible convenience foods. (They contain such a mass of confusing substances that it is often very hard to figure out exactly what may be causing you a problem.)

Keep a food diary

Record any foods which you find you react to negatively and try eliminating them from your meals altogether. Make a note of these in your journal, with the date of the trial, and then stay away from them for a month and test again. As your system gets clearer and stronger from all of the techniques and health-enhancing tools you may be introducing into your life, you will probably find you can handle many foods which previously caused you problems.

All this may sound complicated and a bit of a nuisance to work out, but the difference this testing process can make to anyone who experiences food-sensitivity symptoms can be tremendous, both emotionally and physically. And it costs nothing but a little time and effort. Many women who have trouble shedding fat, find that when they identify foods to which they are sensitive and eliminate them, excess fat melts away without their ever having to count a calorie. Also, identifying food sensitivities and eliminating the trouble makers from your diet can raise energy levels dramatically.

Quiz three

☐ Do you eat refined carbohydrates such as bread, cakes, biscuits and pasta made from white flour?
☐ Do you often suffer from abdominal bloating and wind?
☐ Do you suffer from chronic constipation and/or diarrhoea?
☐ Do you have a history of yeast or fungal infections such as vaginal thrush or athlete's foot?
☐ Have you taken antibiotics repeatedly for a persistent infection or skin problem?
☐ Do you take or have you taken a birth control pill for more than 6 months?
☐ Do you suffer from low back pain?
☐ Are you addicted to sugary foods or to alcohol?
☐ Do you suffer from menstrual difficulties – cramping, excessive bleeding, endometriosis?
☐ Do you find the taste of garlic intolerable?

If you answered yes to 5 or more of these questions you might expect a proliferation of Candida. Read on.

The yeast syndrome

The common yeast, Candida albicans, lives harmlessly in the gastrointestinal tract of all of us along with a lot of other micro organisms, some of which, like certain flora in the bowel, actually support high-level health. Candida is the yeast which, if it proliferates in the vaginal tract, can cause thrush. Under certain circumstances Candida overgrowth occurs to produce a complex medical syndrome known as the yeast syndrome or chronic

WHAT DO YOU CRAVE?	
Foodstuffs	**Suspect**
Biscuits, bread, pastry and pasta?	Wheat
Coffee or cola? Do you drink more than 2 glasses a day?	Caffeine
Pizza, tomato sauce, spaghetti?	Tomatoes
Orange drinks, oranges, orange sorbet?	Oranges
Wine?	Grapes, sugar or yeast
Chocolate?	Sugar, chocolate or processed fats
Cheese, butter, yogurt?	Milk
Icecream or creamy desserts?	Milk, sugar or junk fats

candidiasis. The organism has 2 forms, a yeast or blastospore form and a fungal form into which it can turn. The fungal form is capable of penetrating the mucosal cells in the gut and disrupting the absorption of nutrients from the foods you eat. This can lead to proteins in their unbroken-down form (and toxic wastes from the Candida itself) entering the bloodstream via the walls of the intestines. Once there they wreak havoc with your body.

Some common symptoms frequently traced back to overgrowth of Candida in the gut include loss of energy, chronic fatigue, decreased libido, bloating and wind, depression and irritability, inability to concentrate, low immune function (making you susceptible to colds and 'flu) food sensitivities and cravings for foods rich in carbohydrates or yeast.

Some of the situations which encourage the proliferation of

Candida include the taking of broad-spectrum antibiotics and other drugs, the presence of diabetes, eating a lot of sugar, not having sufficient digestive secretions, and taking the Pill. All of these things create an internal environment in your body which encourages this yeast/fungus to burgeon. The medical diagnosis of chronic candidiasis is difficult to make because there is no single specific diagnostic test for it and because many doctors still know little about it. That is the bad news.

The good news is that most of the things you can do to improve the overall quality of your diet such as cutting out junk fats, sugar and highly processed foods (all of which the Candida thrives on) alter the internal environment and discourage the proliferation of this yeast/fungus. If you suspect candidiasis, experts offer the following advice. It is useful to try out what they suggest as it does not contradict the general guidelines for good eating and has made an enormous difference to the lives of many people who unbeknownst to them had been made miserable by this condition:

• **Drop the drugs** Don't take antibiotics, steroids or birth control pills (unless there is a real medical necessity).

• **Change your diet** Avoid refined carbohydrate foods like white flour, refined sugars such as corn syrup and glucose, fruit juices and honey. Avoid milk products and all foods to which you suspect you might be allergic or sensitive. Don't eat foods with a high yeast or mould content such as alcohol, cheese, peanuts, dried fruits and grapes. Eat lots of fresh vegetables (except yams, parsnips, corn and potatoes). Eat as much as you like of fish and game, lamb and whole grains except wheat. Limit the fruits you take to no more than 3 cups a day chosen from apples, berries, pears and bananas.

• **Check for food sensitivities** Food sensitivities are common with Candida. The things you crave are frequently what the yeast itself craves. Try to identify any possible sensitivities and weed them out through changes in diet. This can help a lot.

• **Drink Pau d'Arco** This tea from the South American tree has a long folk use in the treatment of infections probably due to its lapachol content. Both lapachol and other compounds from Pau d'Arco have demonstrated anti-candida effects.

• **Go for help** If these things do not make a significant difference then seek out a doctor who is genuinely knowledgeable about the treatment of Candida. It is not enough

simply to give a fungicidal drug which is the usual treatment. While it can suppress the Candida when you are taking it, often when you stop it regrows so you are soon back where you started. Once the Candida is under control you will probably be able to eat everything you like so long as you continue to steer clear of unnecessary drugs and highly processed foods. But be patient. It takes time for nature to rebalance your body.

Beware the mycotoxins

Grains are a common troublemaker for many women. They can suppress energy, cause weight gain and even contribute to constipation. These symptoms can be the result of a specific grain sensitivity, wheat being the most common culprit. Or they can be a reaction to the mycotoxins in the grains from which our breads and cakes and biscuits and pasta and cereals are made. Mycotoxins are various forms of fungi and moulds with long names like Tremorgans, Aflatoxins and Roridins which, unbeknownst to us, infest most of the grain from which our foods are made. In the past half century, our foods have been stored for long periods in damp conditions because regulations allow moisture to be added to dry grains and dealers can increase profits by adding weight to their stores. Foods also travel long distances. As a result mycotoxins have proliferated almost exponentially. They can be responsible for conditions as different as dermatitis, fatigue, mental confusion and digestive problems. So far very little has been made public about mycotoxins. British expert in the

field Alisdair Tainsh has written extensively on the subject, even linking certain supposed deficiency diseases such as beri-beri to the presence of these fungal nasties in grains. It is worth experimenting with cutting out all grains and cereals from your diet for a fortnight just to see if your health and good looks improve. If you notice a marked difference, you might like to cut them out altogether or to eat them only occasionally, as we prefer to do.

Quiz four

☐ Do you consider yourself overweight?

☐ If so, have you been overweight for more than 5 years?

☐ During the past year have you been on at least one reducing diet?

☐ If you have, has the diet involved limiting the *variety* of foods you eat (as opposed to simply their quantity?)

☐ Do you ever skip meals in an attempt to keep your weight down?

☐ Has your weight fluctuated by more than 10 pounds during the past year?

☐ Do you tend to eat next to nothing during the day and have your main meal late at night?

☐ Do you often feel guilty about what you eat?

☐ Do you ever take artificial appetite suppressants?

☐ Do you take laxatives regularly?

If you answered yes to 5 or more of these questions then you need to take a new approach to weight loss. Helpers on this road are: the elimination of food sensitivities, good food combining and regular aerobic activity. Read on.

Slim or flabby?

Crash diets screw up your body's ecology. They are a dangerous way of trying to attain or hold on to what you think is your ideal weight. We say *think* because a lot of women spend a lot of time and effort trying to fit into somebody else's idea of what weight and body size is best for them. Your body *knows* better than anything or anyone else what is right. If, after listening to it carefully and working through some of the exercises in the earlier chapters, you feel that it is not the shape it is meant to be then you can take steps to do something to change this through exercise and food combining (see Chapter 9, Energy Grazing, and Chapter 10, Energy in Motion). Don't go on to the latest slimming diet or rush out and buy a bag full of so-called diet food. Both can deplete you of minerals essential to fuel your metabolic processes. They can also suppress your metabolism so you grow fat on very little food. Besides, they don't work. Statistics show that 95% of women gain back the weight they have lost on a crash diet within months.

Most slimming diets break down muscle tissue on which firm flesh depends. When you regain the weight, the muscle is replaced by fat and sludge which can turn to cellulite. Crash diets can also upset your blood-sugar regulating mechanism so you suffer energy slumps in the day or chronic fatigue.

Identifying any food sensitivities which may be affecting you and excluding the offending foods from your diet, together with the work alone in your journal and a simple form of food combining, is the best way to help your body readjust its own weight naturally, simply and effectively so that the positive changes last. These steps will also help keep your energy high and your body lean. We recently met a young woman in New Zealand who had shed 6 stone in this way in 6 months without going hungry. Decide right now that *you* matter most and do all you can to support yourself in every way you know how. The result will be a stronger, firmer, more beautiful body that resists degeneration and eliminates once and for all the flab our unnatural food habits in the West can make us prone to.

Quiz five

☐ Do you choose margarine rather than butter?
☐ Are you more than a stone over your ideal weight?
☐ Do you suffer from cellulite?
☐ Do you suffer from skin conditions such as eczema or acne?
☐ Do you regularly eat fried foods such as a fried breakfast, french fries, fish and chips?
☐ Do you find that you crave fatty foods?
☐ Do you eat pre-cooked meals, tinned or convenience foods?
☐ Do you cook with polyunsaturated oils such as corn, safflower, sunflower or groundnut?
☐ Do you use commercial salad dressings, salad creams or mayonnaise?
☐ Do you eat commercial snack foods such as crisps and salted peanuts?

If you answered yes to 5 or more of these questions go back and read carefully the section on PUFAs on p.60. Then read on.

Cut out junk fats

PUFAs in their natural state come in a chemical configuration known as a *cis* form. They are rather like gloves which fit perfectly the 'hands' of the molecular fat receptors in your body. But food processing and the heat that is applied to cooking oils when you fry foods converts these *cis* fatty acids into what is known as *trans* fatty acids.

Such trans fatty acids not only don't fit hand-in-glove into your body's metabolic machinery, their presence in your body actually gums up the works. *Every* processed fat (with which, like sugar, convenience foods are loaded) contains these unhealthy fatty acids. You cannot find one margarine on the market which is genuinely health-promoting, despite all the advertising designed to convince us to the contrary. And don't be misled by the words 'contains polyunsaturates' on the label. Margarines and almost all of our cooking oils contain massive proportions of these health-undermining trans fatty acids, whose presence can not only prevent your body from getting the essential PUFAs it needs for health, but can actually block the uptake of any cis fatty acids in good healthy foods you may be eating as well. As a result, although almost half of the calories we consume come from fat, our streets are full of men and women walking around with essential fatty acid deficiencies. (See p.99 for information about good fats.)

Quiz six

☐ Do you live in a city?

☐ Is your home underneath or near electricity pylons?

☐ Do you regularly spend time sitting in traffic or do you walk or cycle near traffic?

☐ Do you drink tap water?

☐ Do you eat foods cooked in aluminium or copper-lined cooking pots?

☐ Do you smoke several cigarettes per day or spend at least an hour a day in the company of smokers?

☐ Do you eat fruits and/or vegetables without washing them?

☐ Do you spend more than 2-3 hours in front of a VDU per day?

☐ Do you eat out in restaurants at least 3 times a week?

☐ Do you have more than 6 silver amalgam fillings?

If you have answered yes to more than 5 of these questions then you need to take action to decrease the amount of environmental stressors you are exposed to and improve the quality of your home and workplace. Read on.

Scan the environment

Just as we have messed up our food's ability to nourish us at the highest levels for health, so have we interfered with our environment in ways that deplete energy and undermine health. Electromagnetic pollution, heavy metals such as lead and aluminium in our foods, and chemical pollutants in the buildings we live and work in, can all in different ways interfere with your body's metabolic processes on which the production of energy for life depends.

Take a good look at where you are living and working and see what needs improvement. Do what you can to make your environment more health-supporting in every way – by not drinking tap water for instance. Not only are there many harmful chemicals in the water, the chlorine itself is dangerous. An American study has shown that serum cholesterol levels in both men and women are significantly higher in areas with chlorinated water compared to non-chlorinated areas. Be aware that plastics put in a microwave oven, even if declared safe by manufacturers, can give off harmful chemicals that contaminate your food and air. Throw out aluminium pans and replace them with stainless steel or enamelled cookware. Stay away as much as possible from polluted air. Learn as much as you can about the negative effects of exposure to rays from VDUs and chemical solutions regularly used in workplaces. Then educate your bosses and help them take action to improve things. There are studies which show that installing good air-purifying equipment, full-spectrum lighting, ionizers and protection from VDUs can more than make up for the cost of these things in lowered absenteeism and work productivity. Consider using a magnetic bed which produces a negative magnetic field (see Chapter 11, Feeding the Core).

Chapter 8

Passage *to* power

Examining what works in your life and what doesn't takes courage. It is never easy. It demands that you unscramble structures that you take for granted but which may no longer serve you at the deepest level. These can include anything from a habit of munching your way through two pounds of chocolates every time you feel depressed, to holding on to a job that is meaningless, or to a relationship which does not help you grow – all because you are afraid you can't cope otherwise or do any better for yourself.

Metamorphosis for freedom

Every transformation, every profound and life-enhancing change in some way involves *dismemberment*. It dissolves every structure that has become inadequate to support an organism. Like the crab which sheds his cramped shell in order to create a larger one, each of us again and again is faced with the prospect of taking apart structures in our own lives which have become too small to contain us. If we don't *consciously* rise to the occasion, then life takes them apart for us and we find ourselves precipitated into crises. It seems as though you have entered a dark tunnel leading to an unknown land. You feel that you don't know yourself any more, or what you value, or even what is going on. So fundamental is this uncomfortable but necessary process of *moulting* to human physical, emotional and spiritual health – in fact to life itself – that it takes place again and again in our lives whether we like it or not.

Sometimes change comes spontaneously as a result of something that happens to us – the death of a loved one perhaps, or the loss of a job. Sometimes it is consciously chosen out of an awareness that our current life structures no longer serve our values and our goals. Whether the transition required is a big one (choosing to enter or leave a long-term relationship) or a relatively small one (putting yourself through a short spring cleaning diet to detoxify your body) it frequently brings an experience of deep uncertainty and anxiety – the sense that you are in crisis. The transition facing you seems terrifying. You want most of all to run away. You feel overwhelmed and unable to cope.

The irony in all this is that it is only in facing a crisis and making the transitions it demands that we learn we *can* cope, and that life *can* be trusted. We also discover that, given half a chance, the body has an amazing capacity to heal itself, and that there exists deep within us a wisdom and a clarity more profound and powerful than the conscious mind. The Lebanese poet Kahlil Gibran wisely wrote, 'Your pain is but the breaking of the shell than encloses your understanding.'

For most of us, learning to live through our crises and to make something positive out of them means revising a lot of what we have been taught about ourselves, our minds, even life itself. Most of all it means looking at the concept of crisis and the experience of change from a whole new point of view. It means learning to transform what may feel like a life-threatening situation into a true passage to power.

From crisis to creativity

Christmas had been full of laughter. But on Boxing Day when the children left, Emma began to cry. Grief racked her body. It was as though she had been taken over by a power beyond herself. There was no apparent reason for this yet it went on for three hours. That was the beginning. Within three weeks, each time she went out to walk in the woods near her house, the trees, the grass, the rocks – all came alive. They seemed to vibrate with energy and to glisten with light, almost to breathe. Their colours had become overwhelming – too intense to bear. Panic set in. This healthy and competent woman in her early fifties feared that she was losing her mind. The doctor suggested tranquillizers, sleeping pills and psychotherapy. 'Don't worry,' he assured her, 'we will soon have it all under control.'

For Rebecca, aged 32, the crunch came at work after neglecting her relationship with her lover and ignoring a mounting biological urge to have a child, then passing up two intriguing job offers and working 18 hours a day for 7 months on a marketing plan for a new toothpaste. She knew the plan was just what she needed for a promotion which would make her the first woman on the board. Then the managing director announced the takeover. The launch had to be scrapped. The product would have been in direct competition with the new company's own product already on the market. Two days later her boyfriend announced he had fallen in love with someone else and was leaving. Then one morning while doing her morning run in the park, Rebecca sprained her left ankle so badly that she could not walk at all for two weeks. This meant that now, when it was absolutely crucial that she be at work to secure her future, she found herself completely bedridden. She felt her life collapsing around her and knew she was helpless to do anything about it.

The signs of moulting

Two women in crisis – that moment in life when the foundations of personal safety, beliefs, security or values are challenged overwhelmed by either internal forces or external events. When any one of us experiences such a crisis it is a sign that a moulting is about to take place. We are being asked to walk a passage which, if made with awareness and trust, can expand our experience of life and our sense of ourselves enormously. This demand for personal metamorphosis may be triggered by a death, the ending of a love affair, the recognition that one is addicted to alcohol, drugs or work, a dawning awareness that what you have always worked for and what you have achieved no longer holds meaning for you, the loss of a job or reputation, or even the detoxification process of a cleansing regime. Although each person's metamorphosis is unique, experiences of profound change nevertheless have much in common.

The advice to people in the midst of crisis is pretty standard too. It goes something like this: 'Pull yourself together,' or 'Don't worry,' or 'Go and see the doctor' (who most often supplies a long-standing prescription for potent anti-depressants, barbiturates, or tranquillizers). In the case of women – particularly women of menopausal age – the men in their lives (whether they be husbands, lovers or bosses) are frequently made so uncomfortable by the unexpected changes in a woman's feelings and behaviour (changes that they themselves feel unable to handle) that they insist she must be mentally or biologically ill. For they, like most of us, just want things to return to normal. We are all afraid of crisis and fair enough. Change that is truly transformative seldom comes easily.

Pivots for change

A growing number of biologists, psychologists and philosophers believe that our attitude to crisis needs re-examining. They insist (as the two of us in our own struggles for individual freedom continually discover), that crisis need not be a negative event. Handled positively it frequently portends the unleashing of powerful creative energies. Instead of taking tranquillizers and battening down the hatches when your life seems to be falling apart, it can be useful to begin looking at crisis as a *pivot for change* – a door to the kind of transformation the caterpillar undergoes. Deeply woven into the silk threads of his cocoon, the creature's body dissolves into white jelly only to be reformed again in a completely different shape and set free as a butterfly.

Of course old attitudes die hard. Most psychologists and physicians still see things as Freud did. They still believe that the unconscious mind is full of dangerous repressed impulses and material that, if you are to remain balanced and healthy, you need to keep the lid on. Freud's assertions, brilliant though they were, were a product of the nineteenth century mechanistic thinking on which he was raised. Freud completely ignored the spiritual dimension of consciousness, believing that such phenomena as visions of angels and devils were *always* an indication of pathology.

For half a century other psychiatrists and psychologists – from Carl Jung (who formulated the concept of the Self, the archetypal unchanging centre which has both universal and individual characteristics) to Abraham Maslow, who first coined the phrase 'peak experience' and Roberto Assigioli, who is responsible for the concept of the *higher self* – have insisted that Freud's model of the mind, like the worldview out of which it developed, is too limited.

These men have been instrumental in the formation of new paradigms of consciousness which take in the spiritual dimension of human life. They no longer view the human mind as a static entity, the balance of which must be maintained at all costs. They see each of us involved in a constant process of spiritual growth and a movement towards wholeness. The twists and turns through which we pass in life, they say, are part of this movement, and each crisis – each moulting – is an attempt to bring us closer and closer to being able to live from our own centre and experience our own wholeness. Metamorphosis should not be viewed as something to be avoided, they say. It is as common and as natural as birth, growth, death – part of existence.

Transpersonal perspectives

Such a notion has long existed in religious spheres and is echoed in Biblical phrases such as the process of 'becoming what thou art' but was completely new to psychology. This new view of consciousness not only recognizes the conscious mind, of which we are aware in our day-to-day life, and the unconscious mind, which directs the basic psychological activities and instinctual urges and which encompasses archetypal energies, but also what is often referred to as the *super-conscious* or *transpersonal* mind. The transpersonal realm is described as the domain of higher feelings and capacities including intuition and inspiration. It is called transpersonal because it is more than personal. It also taps universal consciousness crossing over barriers of culture to connect us with the universal energies.

The acknowledgement of the transpersonal realm by psychologists closely parallels findings in the new physics which emphasize both the interconnectedness of all life and the all pervasive stuff of consciousness. Often a woman undergoing a major crisis finds she has tapped into this universal consciousness and is experiencing other dimensions of being or even other times and places. When this happens, it can bring about quantum leaps in personal growth and creativity. It is then that crisis becomes transformational.

Mid-life transition

Take the case of Emma. Her background was simple. After many years as a successful wife and mother she approached the time in her life when all of the structures on which her life had been built were becoming redundant. Her children had left home for university and work. Her husband, the managing director of a large engineering firm, travelled a lot and she, who had given up a job in publishing twenty five years before to look after her young family felt she had little to look forward to. Before crisis struck, Emma had become vaguely aware of these things and told herself she should take up a hobby or go back to work but nothing grabbed her interest. Thanks to the success of her husband's business, she did not need to earn money. When unable to cope with the strange states of consciousness into which she found herself plunged, and on the advice of friends and family, she sought help from the doctor, he told her she was menopausal and wrote out a prescription for tranquillizers and hormone replacement. Something prevented her from having the prescription filled. 'I feared I was losing my mind and I was absolutely terrified that these intense visual experiences together with sensations of powerful energies flowing through my body in waves day after day were a sign that I was actually going to die,' she says, 'but a small voice somewhere deep inside me kept saying "see it through – don't run away from it." I didn't know where to turn. Everyone, including my husband, thought I was irresponsible not to do as the doctor advised. The irony was that the one thing I had always prided myself on was my sense of responsibility.'

The healing power of friendship

As it turned out Emma was lucky. Despite her embarrassment and shame about what had been happening to her, she frequently spoke about it to people whom she did not know very well. 'It was as if I had to tell someone,' she says, 'and I couldn't speak to my family and closest friends since they were convinced I was crazy.' One of the people she told was a woman who had herself been through a similar experience five years earlier. Emma, relieved to find anybody who 'understood' and didn't brand her psychotic, began spending time with this woman.

On the advice of her husband, who thought a change of scene would be good for her, she decided to spend a fortnight with her new friend in a small holiday cottage in the Lowlands of Scotland. There the two women lived together, ate together and walked in the wilderness. Emma's symptoms continued but the woman she was with was not in the least afraid of them, neither did she worry about Emma's intense emotions – feelings of grief at the loss of her children, of uncertainty about her future, of abandonment much like a baby must feel when taken from its mother – nor about her strange bodily sensations which were particularly severe at night. She simply stayed with her friend and *allowed* it all to happen. In Emma's own words, 'The experience of her simply letting me be in the state I was in and her complete sense of trust that what was happening to me was all right was incredible for me. I learnt from it that the death I feared was not physical death as I had thought but the death of everything in myself that was *meant* to die – the end of the life I had lived as a mother, always sacrificing myself for the sake of my children and my husband, and the death of my image of myself as a responsible but limited person with no real sense of identity apart from the way I could serve others.'

After about ten days her symptoms peaked and then began to subside. By the time she got home she was still experiencing strange energy flows in her body and the colours still seemed extraordinarily bright (it took about three months for all that to change) but now she no longer feared what was happening because, she says, 'I could feel for the first time in my life that there really was something inside me – something very alive and real. I am determined to get to know it and to find out what it is all about. Where it will lead I don't know. I have begun to paint – to try to get some of that vibrancy of colour on paper. Incidentally, a lot of people

don't like the "new me". They prefer the "good old reliable Emma". But I feel, far from my life being over, that I am beginning a new adventure and that wherever it takes me, it is uniquely mine.'

Harbingers of change

This sense of impending death which Emma experienced is common in the experience of moulting. It is something Leslie has experienced again and again before a major change takes place in her life. As American expert in transformative psychology John Wier Perry MD says, 'Whenever a profound experience of change is about to take place, its harbinger is the motif of death. This is not particularly mysterious, since it is the limited view and appraisal of oneself that must be outgrown or transformed, and to accomplish transformation the self-image must be dissolved… one is forced to let go of old expectations… let oneself be tossed about by the winds of change…cultivating a more capacious consciousness, open to new dimensions of experience.'

Perry, a Jungian analyst, encourages people to work through their experiences – even when they are very extreme – without the mitigating effect of drugs. Instead they are given the support of a safe place to be while their particular moulting is taking place and a lot of loving support from people who have, from experience in their own lives, learned to turn the experience of crisis into a passage to power. Perry insists that, like the crab in need of a new shell, what precipitates such a crisis is the surfacing of energy from deep within the psyche which has been bound up in the structures of a self-image or a worldview that has become obsolete – too limited to suit a person's needs.

Where inner and outer meet

One of the most common objections amongst conventional 'batten-down-the-hatches' psychologists to viewing crisis as part of a transformational process is that while a crisis such as Emma's appears largely to have arisen from within, that of Rebecca was triggered entirely by outside events – the company takeover, the decision of the man in her life to leave her, the accident to her ankle which put her to bed – all things over which she had no control. Or was it? According to British transpersonal psychologist Barbara Sommers, the outer and the inner world are not as separate as we might imagine. A woman like Rebecca may be far more responsible for precipitating the outer events that triggered her crisis than she thinks.

Each of us has an inner and an outer world. When these two get out of balance, say, by emphasizing external or material values to the detriment of more personal deeper values, then a person invites disruption. The more someone like Rebecca pushes on with her ambitions and neglects her inner voice, the closer she brings herself to situations that precipitate crisis. Then crisis becomes a way of rebalancing things by forcing her to turn and look within.

Things fail: she loses the man she loves because she has, by her actions, undervalued and neglected the relationship and she damages her body so she is quite literally *forced* to go to bed, to be alone and to listen to her inner voice. In Sommers' words, 'The real woman inside her doesn't like the way she has been living so she starts to cry out, "What about me?" The more she drives her energy into her conscious external life, the more power from her unconscious is generated to redress the balance. The "feeling" side of her (as opposed to the "doing" side) actually *magnetizes* a field around her so things start to happen.' According to Sommers the important thing about Rebecca's crisis is that out of its forcing her to *be* with herself instead of constantly being caught up in *doing* comes the opportunity to ask questions such as 'Who am I?' and 'What do I want? – is my goal really to have a seat on the board? Or is that something I think I want because my father, my society, my friends think it is important?'

Rehearsal for change

All crises big or small are opportunities to get in touch with the wholeness of ourselves not just to live lopsidedly or as partial people pushed into the way we are living by our culture, by education or by other people's views or values.

All crisis offers transformation provided, as the poet Relke says, we have the courage to embrace it: '…this very abyss is full of the darkness of God, and where one experiences it, let him climb down and howl in it (that is more necessary than to cross over it).'

Open your journal and look back to the first few pages where you have answered the questions: 'Who are you?', 'What do you want?' 'Where are you now in relation to what you want?' and finally, 'What do you *think* is stopping you?' First ask yourself if any of your original answers to the questions have changed? If so

record the changes (or additions) in your journal. Then, in the light of the information in the last three chapters, let yourself become aware of any structures in your own life – emotional, physical, environmental, intellectual – which no longer serve you and the choices you are making. See if there are any passages which are appropriate for you to make consciously. Making simple changes *willingly* can be useful practice for developing the skill of transforming crises, when they appear, into passages to power.

You might like to experience the passage to new energy clarity that a detoxification diet followed for a few days can bring. (You'll find such a regime in the next chapter.) Or you might try doing without some addictive substance or activity which you feel is draining your energies. If you choose to do either, notice any changes that come about and pay attention to any messages that you get from within in the process.

If during any passage you find yourself temporarily faced with a feeling of the blues or hopelessness (descending into an internal state which we call Dismal Swamp), you will find some suggestions of external and internal techniques in the next chapter which we have found helpful in making some of our own transitions. Your endless energy journal can be of great help too. Get into the habit of recording new insights that come with change. They can serve as the foundation for the new structures you need to build so that in time every crisis can become a passage to power.

Workbook *for* Passage *to* power

The transition towards a lifestyle which fully honours core energy can be difficult. While each step you take towards living from your core brings you more energy and greater freedom, it also requires that you let go of energy-draining attitudes or habits. When these habits are things you have relied upon for years, giving them up – no matter how attractive the reward – can be like pulling teeth from a hippopotamus. Just as an addict may have to go through a painful process of withdrawal before becoming free of the addiction, so you may have to brave a few unpleasant healing or cleansing reactions if you are fully to access your personal power and endless energy.

What do we mean by healing or cleansing reactions? A cleansing reaction can be anything from a physical symptom such as a headache, when your body begins to clear waste rapidly, to a depression or spiritual crisis as you delve within the depths of your soul in an attempt to discover meaning and reorientate your life. Far from trying to sidestep such reactions, we have learnt whenever possible it is better to meet them head on. When you can, they invariably lead you into a new realm of energy and wellbeing. This is not to say we enjoy cleansing reactions – no one does. But with a little trust, and some useful self-help techniques (see A Helping Hand and Navigating Dismal Swamp), it is possible to ride the wave of healing reactions with relative ease and move from crisis to creativity.

We all have blocks – physical, emotional and psychological which build a wall between where we are now and where we would like to be. Every conscious choice you make to honour your core – whether it be to get in touch with your instincts through movement or to take time each day to care for the way you look – chips away a little piece of the blocks that make up your wall. And each chip out of the wall brings you a little closer to your own power. Some choices, such as the choice to take up regular exercise, may have more impact than others. One that is particularly helpful in encouraging the breakthrough to power is the choice to do a cleansing diet. If you are keen to experiment with the process of change and encourage a passage to power you might like to try the 7 Day Cleanse. In the pages that follow you will also find some techniques which can be helpful when, for one reason or another, you find yourself having to cope with the crisis blues and navigate Dismal Swamp.

7 *day cleanse*

Some of the most rapid energy breakthroughs we have witnessed in ourselves and others have been as a result of a cleansing diet. Although we have used countless such regimes over the years, each time we begin one there is always a sense of great excitement. For each time we commit ourselves to clearing out old wastes and welcoming in vitality we emerge with a fresh outlook on life.

The 7 Day Cleanse makes use of the essential life energy in fresh foods, as well as several amazing natural nutritional 'supplements' such as spirulina, linseeds and mixed fibre. It is designed to last from Wednesday to the following

Tuesday so the most intense cleansing days fall at the weekend, allowing you to rest during them if you feel the need. A short and simple detoxification regime such as this one is generally considered safe for anyone who is not on drug therapy or who is not suffering from liver or kidney disease. But it is always a good idea to check with your doctor – his reassurance can help you relax more and enjoy the process of detoxifying your body. Let's take a look at the Cleanse.

1: Energy boosting
During the first 2 days of the Cleanse (Wednesday and Thursday) you exclude the energy-draining foods, as well as wheat and milk products, and go for energy-enhancers: wholefoods, nutritional supplements, exercise and skin brushing. You encourage elimination of wastes by taking a colon-cleansing supplement – a good fibre complex or psyllium husk powder – twice a day.

2: Raw impact
The third day (Friday) of the Cleanse is a transition into the weekend Power Cleansing. You take the process of elimination a step further by eating only raw foods (the most highly cleansing of all). You also exclude protein, easing the load on your digestive system and helping your body to concentrate on the clearing of wastes. The Raw Impact phase introduces spirulina as a potent cleanser and energizer and uses plenty of sprouted seeds/pulses for their detoxifying properties.

3: Power cleansing
This part of the Cleanse (Saturday and Sunday) gives your body the optimum conditions to throw off wastes quickly and safely. The fibre supplement provides bulk which not only satisfies hunger pangs on this semi-fast, but helps flush wastes out of the colon so that they don't remain in your system to cause cleansing reactions. The spirulina broth maintains energy and blood-sugar levels so that you don't feel weak (p.79). During the Power Cleanse apples or raw carrots are eaten freely to support the cleansing process. The semi-fast is broken on Sunday night with a delicious all-raw salad to help ease you into Energy Maintenance.

4: Energy maintenance
Phase four (Monday and Tuesday) of the Cleanse eases you back into your normal way of eating. It is the same as the 'Easing in' Energy Booster, days 1 and 2. It provides your body with optimal energy foods which can be incorporated into your regular way of eating to create your own high-energy foodstyle. The fibre routine can be continued twice a day to help keep your colon clean until you use up your supplement supply. Similarly, the other components of the cleanse, from spirulina to skin brushing and exercise can also become part of your daily routine.

The cleanse

Before you start the 7 Day Cleanse, gather the items you will need. Order the special supplements well ahead of time. The weekend before your chosen week begin to grow your sprouts (see p.97 for help). Stock your larder with the items suggested from the health food store. On the Monday or Tuesday

- **Spring water** 7 one-litre bottles – 1 to be drunk daily between meals to encourage elimination.
- **Herbal teas** Simple teas such as peppermint, fennel or liquorice are ideal for an upset stomach. Or try a flavourful blend. Choose a selection of teas to tempt your taste buds and be sure to steep them well for flavour (see Resources, p.137 for some of our favourites).
- **Honey** for sweetening your herb teas if needed.
- **Protein** selections for days 1 and 2...6 and 7. For non-vegetarians/vegans: free-range eggs, free-range poultry, organically raised meat (such as lamb's liver), fish such as salmon, mackerel, trout, bass.
For vegetarians/vegans: almonds or other unsalted nuts and seeds for salads (see above), tofu, soya milk (without added sweeteners).

From the greengrocer

- **Fresh fruit** in season such as apples, pears, bananas, grapes, berries, melon, etc. (NB If you suspect a Candida problem it is best to avoid eating too much fruit, especially the soft high-sugar content fruits such as grapes, peaches and plums. To discover whether Candida is a problem for you do the quiz on p.66).
- **Fresh vegetables** for salads such as spinach, lettuce (cos, lamb's, radicchio, salad bowl, Chinese leaves), red/white cabbage, watercress, mustard and cress, carrots, beetroot (raw), radishes, turnips, chicory, fennel, red, yellow and green sweet peppers, cauliflower, broccoli, avocados, spring onions, mangetout, french beans, tomatoes, cucumber, courgettes, celery, mushrooms.

- **Other vegetables** for cooking such as potatoes, corn on the cob, parsnips, aubergines, asparagus, green beans, artichokes. (NB If you have a centrifuge juicer and want to make use of the fresh squeezed vegetable juice option during the Cleanse you will need to stock up on suitable juicing material. We recommend carrot juice or carrot mixed 2:1 with apple.)

Salad morsels (optional)

Although as a rule we don't eat convenience foods, we like to keep a few tins (without preservatives) of certain foods that make a nice addition to salads. Some examples are artichoke hearts, hearts of palm, olives, tuna in brine.

Special supplements

These may be bought from your health food store or through mail order (see Resources, p.136-7).

- **Spirulina powder** a natural food supplement made from a special type of algae that is packed with minerals and high-quality protein. (For spirulina's impressive nutritional value, see p.101)
- **Vegetable bouillon powder** the reduced salt variety (also available from some health-food stores) makes a wonderful seasoning for salads and soups. Combine with spirulina powder to make the delicious spirulina broth.
- **Fibre complex** including psyllium, flaxseed, pectin, Lactobacillus acidophilus, Agar Agar and Alginate; or simple psyllium husks (see Resources, p.137). When taken with liquid these supplements expand and form a bulk in the intestines which cleans out mucus, heavy metals and

other waste particles that have accumulated. In some cases such wastes can cling to the colon wall for years, clogging the digestive tract and preventing the absorption of vital nutrients.

Sea plant complex

Sea plants are rich in the minerals which your body's metabolic processes require to function properly. In a time when our foods are becoming increasingly depleted of important minerals and trace elements the use of plants from the sea becomes more and more important. Even things which your system requires in minute quantities such as vanadium, chromium and lithium are found in sea plants. Taking a good supplement can help fill in any mineral gaps. (See Resources, p.137)

Other items

- **A juicer** (optional) for making fresh vegetable and fruit juices.
- **Dry skin brush** made of natural bristles for skin brushing – from chemists or department stores.
- **A food processor or blender** If you don't have one, try to borrow one during the cleanse.
- **Epsom salts** household grade. You will need 500g for 2 elimination baths.
- **Braun Multipractic** (optional). This superb, simple and inexpensive electric mixer comes with its own mixing container. It is particularly useful for preparing the spirulina broth, psyllium mixture, and some breakfasts and dressings.
- **An easy-to-wash cocktail shaker** or screw top jar for the fibre routine.

before you begin, choose your fresh fruits and vegetables as well as the appropriate fresh protein foods you will need.

Use your Endless Energy journal during the Cleanse to record how you feel – not just physically, but emotionally and mentally too. Let it help you gain perspective and clarity as you clear away wastes. Notice if you have a different outlook by the end of the Cleanse.

Days one and two

From here on exclude the following throughout the 7 days:
● **All processed and convenience foods.**
● **All grains** (except sprouted wheat) including bread, pasta, cereals, cakes, biscuits, etc.
● **All dairy produce** including milk, cheese, butter, yoghurt.
● **All stimulants** such as coffee, tea, alcohol, cigarettes.
● **Sugar and artificial sweeteners** – sweets, chocolate, chewing gum.

First thing
The fibre routine. Mix 1 heaped tsp of fibre complex or psyllium powder into 8 fluid ounces of spring water. The best way to do this is to combine the two in a cocktail shaker or screw-top jar and shake to blend. Drink immediately from the container before the mixture becomes too gel-like. Then follow with a chaser of a glass of spring water or a cup of herb tea. You can also use the multipractic to blend combine the water and fibre, but wash it immediately as the mixture quickly gets hard to remove.

Now is an excellent time to take your 30 minutes of aerobic exercise. Aerobic exercise is one of the very

best ways to rid your body of waste, making you look and feel great. If you are not particulary athletic, don't panic. The exercise can be as simple as walking for 30 minutes. Other good choices might be cycling, jogging, rebounding or swimming. (See Chapter 10, Energy In Motion.)

After exercising we make use of one of the old faithful detoxification techniques we have used for years – skin brushing. Skin brushing improves circulation, increases lymphatic drainage and encourages the elimination of toxins through the skin. It is simple and quick and leaves your skin beautifully smooth and glowing. Before your bath or shower, take a natural bristle brush and rub it over the entire surface of your skin (excluding your face and neck). Begin with the soles of your feet and travel up your legs, over your hips and across your back. Use a circular clockwise motion over your abdomen and breast area. Rub from your hands, up your arms and across your shoulders. Then take your bath or shower.

Breakfast
Choose one of these breakfasts.
● Carob Whip: Chop a banana into a bowl. Stir or blend 1-2 table-spoons of Carob Mix into 1/2 a cup of soya milk. Pour the mixture over the bananas and enjoy. To make Carob Mix (enough for several breakfasts), blend 6 tablespoons of linseeds finely in a food processor, then add and blend 6 tablespoons of sunflower seeds and 6 table-spoons of carob powder. You can keep the mixture for a few days in an airtight container in the fridge.
● Fresh Fruit Delight: Grate an apple and/or pear, add a few

berries (optional) and sprinkle with lemon juice. Top with Three Seed Mix and a pinch of cinnamon (optional). To make Three Seed Mix, place 6 tablespoons each of sunflower, pumpkin and sesame seeds in a frying pan and roast them lightly (the roasting is optional, but it brings out their flavour). When the seeds become golden, blend them finely in a food processor. Add 1-2 tablespoons of this mix to your fruit, as well as 1 tablespoon of finely ground linseeds. Keep the extra in an airtight container for breakfasts or to sprinkle over salads.
● Almond Milk Shake: Soak a handful of almonds overnight in a bowl of water. In the morning, drain the almonds and blend them well with a glass of fresh spring water and a few drops of vanilla essence (optional). Add some fruit such as strawberries, raspberries, blackberries or blackcurrants, plus 1 tablespoon of finely ground linseeds. Blend well and sweeten with a teaspoon of honey if desired. Sip and relish.

Mid-morning
● A glass of fresh squeezed carrot juice or a cup of herb tea. An apple if you're hungry.
● Drink from a bottle of mineral water throughout the day, aiming to finish it by bedtime.

Lunch
● A Master Salad including fresh sprouts (see p.92-94). To the salad base add one of the following protein morsels:
● Finely grated hard-boiled egg.
● Some tinned tuna – water packed.
● Tofu dressing (see p.95).
● Toasted nuts/seeds such as pump-kin seeds, cashews or

hazelnuts.
- Sea plant supplement – 3 capsules.

Mid-afternoon
- A glass of carrot juice or a cup of herb tea. An apple if you are hungry.

Dinner
One of the following dishes served with a salad:
- Wok-fried vegetables (see p.93 and 95) served with tofu cubes, or diced chicken breast.
- Omelette cooked in olive oil – either plain or with vegetables such as onion, peppers and mushrooms.
- Baked potato stuffed with Curried Avocado Dip (see recipe, p.95).
- Hearty Vegetable Soup (see recipe, p.96).
- Sprout Burgers (see recipe, p.97).
- Grilled Fish with lemon juice and fresh herbs.
- Lamb's liver sautéed in a little olive oil and chopped onions.
- Sea plant supplement – 3 capsules.

Before bed
- Fibre routine followed by a cup of herb tea.
- Abdominal massage with olive oil. Use a little olive oil to massage your abdomen in a clockwise direction for a few minutes. This encourages the elimination of wastes through the bowel.

Day three
First thing
- Fibre routine and herb tea.
- Exercise and skin brushing.

Breakfast
- Fresh fruit – choose from apples, pears, strawberries, raspberries or other berries – you can use frozen berries if you can't get fresh.

(Bananas are excluded on this day because of their high protein content.)

Mid-morning
- Spirulina broth (or if you don't like the taste of spirulina, 8 spirulina tablets and the broth on its own.) Pour 10 fluid ounces of boiling water into a blender, food processor or Multipractic. Add 1 level tablespoon of spirulina powder and 1 level teaspoon of vegetable bouillon powder. Blend well and drink.

Lunch
- Salad without protein addition but with plenty of sprouts.
- Sea plant supplement – 3 capsules.

Mid-afternoon
As for mid-morning.

Dinner
As for lunch, including sea plant supplement.

Before bed
- Fibre routine and herb tea.
- Abdominal massage.

Days four and five
First thing
- Fibre routine and herb tea.
- Exercise: go for a gentle walk for about 30 minutes now or later in the day. (It's not good to do strenuous exercise during the Power Cleansing days.)
- Skin brushing.
- Wash and scrub a bowl full of carrots and apples to eat whenever you feel like it during the day.

Breakfast
- Spirulina broth or spirulina in juice (carrot or apple juice), or 8

spirulina tablets plus the juice or broth drunk separately.

Mid-morning
- Fibre routine plus water, herb tea or vegetable juice.

Lunch
- Spirulina broth or spirulina in juice, as for breakfast.
- Sea plant supplement.

Mid-afternoon
- Fibre routine plus water, herb tea or vegetable juice.

Saturday dinner
- Spirulina broth or spirulina in juice (as lunch).
- Sea plant supplement.

Sunday dinner
- A large all-raw salad including sprouts but without the protein.
- Sea plant supplement.

Before bed
- Fibre routine and herb tea.
- Abdominal massage.

If you are hungry at any time during the 2 Power Cleanse days you may eat as many fresh raw carrots and/or apples as you like. (Buy organic if possible or wash very well.) Be sure to chew them thoroughly. Include during each of these days a 20-minute detoxifying epsom salts bath (see p.81).

During the Power Cleanse you are particularly likely to experience some form of cleansing reaction, such as fatigue, irritability or a headache. The epsom salts bath helps, but it is also important to lie down and rest if you feel tired. Use the Helping Hand suggestions, p.80, to alleviate specific cleansing symptoms.

Days six and seven

Follow the instructions as for days 1 and 2: Energy Boosting.

A helping hand

When you change your way of eating and provide your system with the best elements to enable it to clear out wastes, you may experience some sort of cleansing reaction. This can be worrying for anyone unaccustomed to the process of elimination. It can lead to mild panic: – 'This new diet can't be doing me any good – I feel awful, I have spots, I have a headache, something's wrong.' Have faith. In a fundamentally healthy person most cleansing reactions will last only a day or two. After that you will begin to feel much better than before and have far more energy. Let's look at how to cope with specific minor difficulties in order to ride the cleansing wave smoothly.

The abdominal compress

This is one of the most effective techniques for helping to eliminate wastes from the body. Many illnesses have their origin in a toxic colon where waste matter accumulates more quickly than it can be got rid of. Applying cold water to the area in the form of a compress charges the local cells with energy, activating circulation and freeing clogged capillaries so that stored wastes can be released more efficiently through the bowel as well as through the skin. A cold compress around the middle may not sound like everyone's idea of fun, but once you have experienced its benefits, you'll become a convert. Not only does it relieve digestive problems, but it is great for insomnia, fever and period pains.

Find a piece of cotton sheeting wide enough to reach from under your arms down to your hips and long enough to wrap around you comfortably. (An old pillowcase ripped open into a long rectangle is ideal.) Dip the cloth into cold water and wring it out. Then wrap it around your middle and secure with safety pins. Wrap a thick dry towel around this and get into a warm bed. You may want to put on a pair of thick socks. It is important that you don't feel cold. Relax for 30 minutes. If you feel like dropping off to sleep for the night you can remove it in the morning.

Morning grouchiness

Anyone who wakes up grouchy is likely to be suffering from an overload of acid wastes in her body. On a cleansing diet this grouchiness is accentuated. Being irritable is no fun for you or anyone around you. The best remedy we have found is a tall glass of freshly squeezed vegetable or fruit juice such as carrot and apple or watermelon. These juices revive the entire body almost instantly by alkalinizing acid wastes. The difference you feel after a fresh vegetable/fruit juice cocktail is remarkable. Another good morning de-groucher is the juice of half a lemon with water and honey.

To bed with fatigue

The only thing we have to say about fatigue as a cleansing reaction is indulge it! Take the phone off the hook, lie down, cover your eyes with an eye mask, stuff your ears with plugs and surrender. If you are tired, but wound up, try the insomnia tips on p.123.

Royal flush for spots

We like to dab a few drops of Tea Tree essential oil onto a spot. It acts as a natural disinfectant and helps blemishes to heal very quickly. A good indication of a toxic colon, spots usually disappear quite quickly as wastes are eliminated. Anyone with a persistent problem might suspect a food allergy (see p.65 for help.) Something we recommend for anyone who has 'tried everything else' to clear up a skin problem is colonic irrigation. One session may be enough, often several are necessary. A rubber tube is inserted into the colon via the rectum and water is flushed in and out to help unblock old waste that has become stuck to the intestinal walls. Sometimes the release of such old stored waste can unblock you in other areas of your life too so that an emotional difficulty can come up to be washed away too.

Of course colonic irrigation is not the most attractive-sounding treatment, and many people are put off by the thought, but for anyone who has suffered the anguish that bad skin can create, it may be worth a try. It is important to encourage the recolonization of helpful intestinal bacteria afterwards by eating live yogurt and taking a pro-biotic supplement.

Headache hints

One of the most common symptoms of rapid elimination is headache. A fabulous hydrotherapy trick to help relieve headache is water stomping. Fill a bath with about 8 inches of hot water. Stomp about in it for about 45 seconds to a minute, then rinse your feet in cool water, dry them well and put on a pair of cosy socks. Lie down and rest for a few minutes with your feet raised 12-18 inches above your head until you feel better.

If you are out and about, try a quick head massage to help clear a headache. Apply pressure with your thumbs to the base of your skull, either side of your spine in line with the bottom of your ears for about a minute. Concentrate on any point that feels particularly tender. Then massage your scalp from your hairline back with all your fingers. For a sinus headache problem, press your thumbs into the inner corners of your eyebrows, just beneath the brow bone, then massage down the sides of your nose and across your cheeks, concentrating on draining away the congestion.

Back out of trouble

Even a backache, which we often assume to be a mechanical problem, can be caused by toxicity in the body. When you begin to eliminate poisons from your body you may experience aches and pains for a day or two. This is just a sign that toxins are being released into your bloodstream ready to be eliminated. Taking a Vitamin C supplement can be very helpful for back or any other aches because Vitamin C encourages the body to release wastes. Choose a supplement without sugar – in powdered or tablet form. Take 1-2 grams every couple of hours until the pain

eases. If this is too much for you, your bowels will simply become loose. Should this happen, cut back on the dose to 'bowel tolerance'. If you suffer from chronic backache, you can do your back muscles a favour by keeping your tummy muscles trim. As the back and stomach muscles work in opposite pairs a slack abdomen means a tight back. Use the Power Toning Routine – in particular Stomach I and II (p.113).

Roll your own spine

If you can't find a masseur, help yourself to a pain-relieving back massage instead. Find a couple of balls the size of a tennis ball. Tennis balls themselves will do, but hollow rubber or plastic children's balls are better because they have more 'give'.

Lie on your back on the floor and place the balls either side of your spine at its base. (If they slip around you can roll them up in a hand towel.) Very slowly roll your body down the balls so that they move up your spine. By bending your knees you can control the amount of pressure you apply. If you come to a spot that is particularly tender, stay still and breathe into it. Imagine releasing any tension with each out breath. When the spot eases, continue rolling. You can work up and down the back several times, easing out any kinks. At the neck use just one ball to roll over the cervical vertebrae. For the upper back and shoulders you can separate the balls, working them over the shoulder blade area. Spinal rolling is particularly beneficial because it stimulates the Chinese acupuncture YU points

which lie either side of the spine and connect with all the body's internal organs. So while you are massaging your back you are also massaging your organs – liver, stomach, colon and heart.

Magical bath salts

For general aches as well as other physical or emotional cleansing reactions, we find nothing beats an epsom salts (magnesium sulphate) bath. Both magnesium and sulphate molecules have an ability to leech excess sodium, phosphorous and nitrogenous wastes from the body. They also have an alkalinizing effect.

Add two cups of household grade epsom salts (available from the chemist) to a bath together with a dessertspoon full of ordinary household bleach (another helper which in *minute* quantities ionizes wastes stored in the body). Fill the bath with warm water and immerse yourself for 20 minutes, topping up with extra hot water.

Emotional healing

The cleansing process not only releases physical wastes but also emotional and psychological ones. It is not uncommon during the Deep Cleanse, for instance, to find yourself mulling over things from your past that you hadn't thought about for years, or letting go of layers of emotional armouring and feeling quite vulnerable. In Navigating Dismal Swamp we will look at helpful ways to handle psychological/emotional difficulties and, in particular, the experience of depression.

The dark journey

When you choose to make a passage to power, or are forced into a crisis situation and want to transform it into a positive experience, you often have to muddle your way through confusion and darkness before things get better. We call this journey navigating Dismal Swamp.

Dismal Swamp is a place you would never choose to go. It is the antithesis to happiness, health and high energy – a place that you would spend any amount of time, energy or money avoiding. Sometimes you can end up in Dismal Swamp without even knowing how it happened. A cloud descends and, before you know it, you find yourself sucked down into the mire of impossibility and depression. Once there, you are forced to wrestle with swamp monsters. These can be anything from fragments of yourself to long forgotten memories or unexpressed feelings. In Dismal Swamp you can only see yourself and your life in the blackest terms.

Over the years we have both come to have an enormous respect for this smelly swamp because within it lies the source of a tremendous amount of energy, creativity and personal power. We find that the more able we are to accept the descent into the swamp when it occurs, and objectively examine the feelings and "creatures" hidden there, the more we can retrieve lost or neglected parts of ourselves in order to emerge with new awareness and an ability to live more fully.

Giving the swamp a place in your life when it comes, however, isn't easy. We are conditioned to believe that 'bad' thoughts or feelings are unattractive and unacceptable. We are taught when we feel down to put on a brave face and snap out of it. Such temporary solutions aren't much help. For when you make a habit of avoiding or suppressing negative feelings you inadvertently feed them with your energy. Then they can become powerful monsters which require increasing amounts of energy to keep at bay. The battle to do so can even make you sick.

Making a passage to power through Dismal Swamp requires objectivity. With a sense of detachment even the most severe depression can become an awakening – an opening to a way of living that is fuller and richer than before. Without objectivity, the most trivial difficulties can plunge you into anxiety or gloom from which there seems no escape.

There are 2 approaches we find helpful. The first involves temporarily embracing the swamp experience. This means consciously choosing to delve into whatever is behind your negative state in order to bring any unconscious or dark area of your psyche to light where it can be worked out. The second approach is to use mind-lifting techniques which enable you to step out of the negative state in order to be able to see what is going on more clearly.

In the midst of any deep change, whether it be physical or psychic or both, you can find yourself submerged in uncomfortable feelings such as hopelessness and despair. Your self-esteem plummets and you feel like poor company. In such a state it is very difficult to take a sympathetic approach – you can *feel sorry for* yourself – but this is not the same thing. Yet to use the Dismal Swamp experience for transformation it is essential to treat yourself with care. Here are 8 reminders to use when you feel yourself slipping into the swamp. They can help you keep your objectivity.

Navigation points

- Acknowledge your right to feel as you do *because* you feel it.
- Approach yourself as you would cradle a newborn kitten in your hands with loving gentleness.
- Be open: listen to your inner self with patience and sensitivity.
- Refuse to judge yourself or say how you should be behaving.
- Accept whatever feelings you have no matter how unworthy they may seem.
- Make a commitment to honour Dismal Swamp and whatever hidden part of yourself may emerge from it.
- Don't identify with the swamp. Dismal Swamp exists as an arena to help you connect with feelings or parts of yourself which may be crying out for attention, but you are not the swamp.
- Keep your sense of humour. A sense of humour is one of the best ways to maintain your objectivity. No matter how awful things may seem, look for the funny side.

Swamp welcome

This exercise counters the 'pull yourself together' approach. It gives you the opportunity to delve beneath the surface of gloom or depression in order to see what may really be going on. It helps you to learn simply to be and to acknowledge all the inadequacies, failings, weaknesses and unpleasant thoughts or feelings you may have with detached indifference. It also promotes an acceptance that is fundamental to personal growth.

Never too low or ugly

The next time you feel down, instead of looking for a temporary solution to escape from your depression, such as alcohol, try getting to the bottom of it instead with this exercise. Begin by sitting or lying comfortably and allow yourself to go deep into the state of Dismal Swamp. Feel the heaviness of the swamp around you. Know that you are safe. Set the scene with whatever murky waters, slime or creeping vines seem appropriate. Gradually allow your thoughts or feelings (about yourself, other people, your life in general) to rise up from the stagnant water.

As the thought arises see it in the form of a swamp creature. So, for instance, if the feeling is, 'I am ugly,' it might be embodied by a dumpy swamp creature covered in warts with a piggy snout, no teeth and no chin. As the creature surfaces, welcome it. Let it announce its essence, 'I am ugly.' You reply, 'Of course you are ugly and you have every right to be ugly, welcome to Dismal Swamp,' then hug the creature and set it on the swamp bank. Prepare to greet the next one, for instance it might be: 'Nothing in my life ever works out.' Allow the creature to emerge and say to it 'I understand that nothing in your life ever works out and you have every right to feel that way.' Then hug the creature and put it on the bank. Another

creature rises up: 'I am angry,' it says. You reply, 'You're angry, I can see that, and you have every right to be angry. I accept and embrace you.' Once again hug it and find it a place on the swamp bank. Continue until each feeling has been given a voice and welcomed with a hug, then thank the creatures from Dismal Swamp. Let the heaviness of the swamp sink into the ground beneath you and lift out of it into ordinary consciousness as you open your eyes.

Swamp dialoguing

The first step to accessing power that has been wrapped up in unconscious thoughts and feelings that may underlie your negative state is giving them an arena in which to feel welcome and accepted. The next step is communicating with them. It may be that in the Swamp Welcome exercise you met one creature who has more energy or more impact than the others. If this is the case, then this particular monster is worth pursuing. Arrange to set up a 'lunch date' on paper. Imagine what that creature would like to eat. Throughout myths or fairytales (the domain of the unconscious) whenever you are dealing with an unfamiliar and potentially destructive creature, it is a safe bet to woo him or her with an offering. The creatures from Dismal Swamp are no exception. Take your pen and journal and let the dialogue unfold…

Swampspeak

Me: Hello Angry Creature from Dismal Swamp – I've brought you some seaweed for lunch.

Swamp Creature: I don't want it.
Me: Why not? I washed it and prepared it for you.
SC: That's the problem – you. You always have to make everything so clean. That annoys me.
Me: Why?
SC: Because I'm messy and you only like clean things.
Me: What would you rather eat?
SC: You.
Me: Why do you want to eat me?
SC: Because I'm angry.
Me: Why are you angry?
SC: Because you don't take me seriously.
Me: How can I take you seriously?
SC: You can give me a place in your life, listen to me and stop doing the things I hate.
Me: Like what?
SC: Like going to dreary dinner parties.
Me: But sometimes I have to go.
SC: Then give me the right to express my anger.
Me: Okay I'll try, but how?
SC: Let me scream.
Me: Feel free.
SC: Aaaarrghh!
Me: Is that better?
SC: A little.
Me: Now would you like some lunch?
SC: Okay, but pass me the slime and grime…

Swamp for swamp

It is important to distinguish between 2 experiences of Dismal Swamp – the swamp as an arena for internal change and transformation, and *swamp for swamp sake*. Sometimes you can get stuck in Dismal Swamp, or in self-pity, re-living the same patterns of negativity on a relentless treadmill that goes nowhere. If you find this happening, it's best to take a break from the swamp.

A good way to recognize swamp for swamp sake is to look out for negative thought patterns. Such patterns, like quicksand, can trap you in the swamp and hinder your passage to power. If you can identify a negative thought pattern you can also help free yourself from it. When you get stuck in Dismal Swamp, ask yourself the following questions:

☐ **Worsifying** Are you exaggerating the importance of a bad event or a mistake you might have made? At the same time are you refusing to recognize or are you belittling your achievements and personal qualities?

☐ **Generalizing** Are you transferring a failing in one area of your life into the belief that you are a failure at everything?

☐ **Condemning** Are you using a single negative event to condemn your future?

☐ **Stringing** Are you supporting a negative belief about yourself by stringing together negative examples from the past?

If you recognize that you are caught in a negative thought pattern and getting nowhere, write your thoughts and feelings down in your journal. Leave it for a few hours and then come back to it. This can give you the objectivity you need to realize just how false a representation of reality your negative thoughts may be.

Stepping out

When the descent into Dismal Swamp takes place in reaction to adverse external events – such as the death of a loved one, a separation, being made redundant or being forced to move home – it can seem like a welcome refuge. Depression provides a buffer to feelings that are too uncomfortable to cope with. If you wallow in the swamp aimlessly for any length of time, however, it can drain your life energy. At this point it is far better to find your way out so that you can deal with your situation and your feelings objectively. Several 'mind lifters' can be helpful.

The mind lifters

We find one of the best ways to step out of the swamp is to do something unexpected that brings you pleasure.

- Bathe in too much bubblebath.
- Dance like a maniac to your favourite old records.
- Play with mud, rocks, clay, dough.
- Eat a salad with fresh flowers in it.
- Draw moustaches on faces in magazines.
- Sing a round with a friend over the phone.

Eat your way free

Whenever either of us sinks to the depths of depression and there doesn't seem to be any particular reason for it – inner or outer – the other will ask 'What have you eaten recently?' It sounds like a rather strange question, but we have found that eating foods that don't agree with us – processed or over-rich foods for instance – can leave us feeling down for no apparent reason. After just a day or two back on a high-raw diet, our biochemical balance is readjusted and we leave Dismal Swamp far behind.

Get moving

Several scientific studies have shown that regular physical activity can help overcome depression and fatigue. An American psychologist, Richard Driscoll, made a study of university students suffering from stress-caused anxiety and depression. Dividing them into groups, he gave one group standard forms of psychotherapy, another drug therapy and made another go running every day. At the end of the term he reassessed the groups and found that the daily runners showed most improvement in symptoms and achieved the highest exam results. Follow-up studies have shown similar results.

Seven blessings

Counting your blessings is an excellent way to turn depression on its head. The next time you feel low, take your journal and make a list of 7 things you have to be grateful for in your life. After counting your blessings, see if you feel any different.

The Bach Remedies

The Bach Flower Remedies, which make use of the encoded structural information in plant essences, are one of the most effective natural ways to help re-establish emotional harmony. They come in the form of tinctures, a few drops of which are placed directly under the tongue or added to a glass of water to be sipped throughout the day. They can be used for chronic (constitutional) or acute emotional imbalances. Three are particularly helpful for Dismal Swamp: Mustard, Gorse and Willow.

Part three

Breakthrough

High-level wellbeing brings an experience of harmony and grace to a woman's life. It helps her live authentically from her core allowing her to call on her own brand of endless energy. It brings a sense of trust…

in herself…

in life…

in the connections between…

all things…

Chapter 9

Energy grazing

Being healthy means a lot more than just not being sick. It means experiencing a sense of grace in your life. It means feeling at *ease*. It means having access to *all* of your being – your imagination, your intellect, your physical strength, and your ability to connect with the world around you through your senses. You sometimes encounter this grace in well-fed young children – children who have been raised on breast milk then given simple wholesome fruits and vegetables, grains and homemade protein foods right from the table. Such a child does not have to stop and consider what she is eating. Provided her taste buds have not been distorted by junk food and processed drinks, she will quite naturally be guided by her own sense of pleasure and preference and will choose the foods she fancies and therefore the foods her body needs. This child is a natural *energy grazer*.

The grace of wellbeing

Studies carried out with small children in such circumstances have shown that, provided the only foods offered them are good foods – that is not highly processed or filled with refined sugar, white flour or additives – children will instinctively choose a wholesome diet. Such a child may eat nothing but bananas one day, then turn to carrots or whole grain bread or eggs the next. Looked at over a period of a week or two, his picking and choosing out of internal, instinctual prompting, spontaneously selects a diet which is virtually ideal when measured against what nutritional science says a growing child needs. Such a child is unconsciously in touch with her body and its needs. She would never give a thought to living from her core. She doesn't have to. She just does it the same way a bird sings or a waterfall tumbles over rocks down into a pool a hundred feet below – each fulfilling its own nature with perfect grace.

The same kind of grace is present when *you* are healthy and whole. There is a sense of trust in yourself, a sense of real connection with the outside world and with the earth, an excitement day to day about your life and what you are going to do next. When what you eat day after day, year after year, supports the energy-balancing, energy-producing processes in your body it helps create an experience of grace in your life. When on the other hand your diet is made up of highly processed foods, filled with junk fats and chemical additives, having lost the complex synergy in all living things – you create metabolic confusion and energy-depletion. This can take you far away from the experience of grace.

What kind of foods best support your core energy? Foods which your own body in its infinite wisdom *desires* when you are experiencing natural balance and grace. Then, like the child, you need give little thought to what is *good for you* – you can simply choose your foods spontaneously, trusting your own instincts as a natural energy grazer. The question for most of us with our hectic lives and pasts filled with processed foods is 'How do I get from here to there?' Some basic principles about eating for good health can be useful in making the transition.

21st century nutrition

When it comes to foods for high-level wellbeing and emotional balance there is one basic principle to remember: *The whole is greater than the sum of its parts.* The best foods are *whole* foods – fresh, natural foods – not foods which have been processed to death. Whole foods have not had every nutrient refined or processed out of them, neither do they come swimming in syrup or emulsified in junk fats. They arrive on your plate and enter your body just as Mother Nature intended them for eating – radiant with their own natural colours and textures and brimming with a complexity of *structural information* essential for maintaining a healthy body and balanced mind. Just what is structural information? It is something you will find mentioned in few books on nutrition. Yet an understanding of it lies at the crux of eating for energy.

The term structural information was coined by an eminent Russian scientist (winner of the much coveted Lenin Prize for Science), Izrail Brekhman of the Far East Academy of Sciences in Vladivostock. He uses it to describe the infinitely complex synergistic, energetic and chemical *order* in living plants and animals on which other living things must feed if they are to maintain high-level health.

According to the Second Law of Thermodynamics the quantity of energy in the world remains constant. This important law of physics is often described as the law of *entropy* – a measure of *disorder* at molecular and atomic levels. Roughly it states that energy in everything is constantly degraded from a higher to a lower order. Gradually, over time, in any system all motion comes to a standstill. Differences in electric or chemical potentials are equalized so that finally a permanent state is reached and the whole system fades into an inert lump of matter. This entropic process of degradation is what you see happen in your garden when a nail rusts. If left there long enough in the wind and the rain and the sun, the nail eventually disintegrates, losing its original form and becomes part of the earth again. It returns to a state of thermodynamic equilibrium or what physicists call *maximum entropy*.

Lifepower

Living systems, like your body, defy this law. So long as your body is alive it is able to avoid decaying into an inert state of equilibrium by assimilating energy from outside through eating for instance. The very high order of the sun's own electromagnetic energy is converted by plants through photosynthesis into material form and stored in enormously complex ways. This life *information* is taken into the plant and embodied in its wholeness. In effect it becomes part of the plant's structure. Then the plant (or an animal who has fed on the plant) brings to the person who eats it a high degree of structural information – the living energetic order which makes us able to resist entropy.

Nobel Laureate physicist Erwin Schrodinger called this process *drinking order* from our environment. To stay healthy – in physical terms for your body to resist degradation or the process of entropy – each of us has to *drink* a lot of *order* – to take into our bodies high-quality structural information via the water we drink, the air we breathe, the electromagnetic fields we are subjected to and, perhaps most important of all, the foods we eat. (By the way, even the thoughts you think and the people you spend time with offer you either more or less drinking order.) When the quality is poor – when they carry more disorder than order – health, clarity of mind, and emotional balance all suffer.

The synergy of energy

As Brekhman says, not only are nutrients which can be measured chemically – vitamins, minerals, protein, etc – important for health, so is the complexity of the way they and other as yet unidentified factors are combined in a particular food as well as the quality of subtle energies the food carries. When we eat natural foods which have been highly processed, fractionated, or filled with chemical additives, we deprive ourselves of their structural information. It has become degraded or destroyed. Such foods no longer carry the ability of this natural order to sustain our lives at a high level of order themselves. For processing foods drastically reduces and disrupts the structural information and a food's health-supporting properties. Eating such foods year after year can steadily degrade the natural order of your body. It creates a seedbed for degeneration, early ageing and illness, and contributes to the kind of mental and emotional imbalance which has become endemic among the youth in our society who have been raised on junk foods.

Drink order

Foods grown on healthy, organic soils and eaten as close as possible to their natural state offer the highest quality structural information. This energy-cum-chemical information all wrapped together in perfect natural synergy enables your body, in Schrodinger's words, *to drink the order it needs* to support core energy. Eating this way gradually lifts your experience of well-being to the highest possible level.

Tell this to the average nutritionist and he will wonder what on earth you are talking about. Most scientists working in the field of nutrition and dietetics are still immersed in the mire of single-cause-single-effect nineteenth-century thinking. They are unconsciously ruled by an outmoded worldview which thinks that what good eating is all about is getting minimum daily requirements of calories, protein, vitamins and minerals, no matter where they come from. Such an outmoded approach to food serves certain commercial interests very well. They would love you to believe that a greasy hamburger on puffy white bread filled with chemicals is every bit as good as one you can make yourself at home with natural foods, given that it contains the same quantity of protein. One fast-food chain not long ago distributed thousands of leaflets all over the world full of bogus nutritional 'information' about how good for you their burgers and fries are. Don't be deceived.

Power foods

To give you some idea of how the health-promoting capacity of food goes far beyond its content of vitamins, minerals, protein and so forth, it can be interesting to look at a vegetable or two and see how many of their

other constituents can be health supporting too. Look up broccoli in a standard book on nutrition for example. It will list a lot of vitamins and some minerals the vegetable contains. What it won't tell you is that this humble member of the brassica family also contains 33 compounds from chlorophyll to vanillic acid which have been shown to have cancer-prevention properties. Or take a look at the humble carrot which has 42, whole oats which contain 18, grapes with 24, and the fresh herb tarragon which in its wholeness boasts an amazing 72 anti-cancer compounds. Such factors go completely unrecognized by run-of-the-mill nutritionists. Yet, like a plant's subtle energies, they play an essential role in the structural information which natural, whole plant foods offer for endless energy. And this kind of analysis doesn't even *begin* to consider the complexity and the synergy of how these ingredients are bound together let alone examine the *energetic* aspects of the structural information the broccoli or the carrot has created for us when it converted the sun's energy through photosynthesis. (Cancer-protective compounds, by their very nature, are also protective against other forms of degenerative conditions – including early ageing.) It only scratches the surface of what both chemically and energetically is present in terms of structural information for high-level health in whole foods grown on soils rich in organic matter.

You can read a hundred books on nutrition – or a thousand – study the interactions of nutrients and the effects of various forms of fat or proteins on cholesterol or triglyceride levels, and even memorize the numbers of calories in every known brand of crackers. But none of it will take you anywhere as close to eating really well as the simple principle: *choose fresh whole foods grown in healthy soils and eat them as close as possible to their natural state.*

Once you get into eating this way you will be on your way to becoming a natural energy grazer. Your body in its balanced wisdom will start letting you know what it needs and you will know that its wisdom can be trusted. That is the grace of wellbeing.

Break all the rules

In food preparation for endless energy it is not *rules* that matter. It is a kind of *affection* towards the foods you choose which is reflected in the affection you feel towards the planet and towards all life. This affection leads you to make certain choices instead of others in food preparation. In fact the affection itself becomes a kind of inspiration. If two things *look* good together they *taste* good together. You wouldn't put octopus and chicken in the same dish for instance. In India the best foods are often those you buy in the cheapest cafés because they have been made with love and joy (and often with humour too). The word café is really a euphemism. For these places are little more than a few stone slabs within which a fire has been built to cook food. Yet the foods they sell are infinitely better tasting, more nourishing and 'safer' than all the fancy foods you get in expensive restaurants. We believe it doesn't matter how skilful, knowledgeable or 'important' a cook is, if she doesn't invest the food she prepares with affection. And care cannot be faked or covered up with skill. Food made without love is *dead*.

Make each meal you prepare, even a simple bowl of yogurt, an adventure. Don't fall into boring habits with food by eating the same thing over and over, or by eating in the same place from the same bowls or plates. If the sun is shining on the landing then take a tablecloth and eat there. Eat in your bed. Eat in a child's room when one of your children is unwell. As often as you can, eat in the open air. If you travel, take a simple

EAT FOR ENDLESS ENERGY

● Choose the foods you prepare for your meals from the best, freshest you can buy on the market (or better still from those grown in your garden or on your windowsill).

● Choose organic vegetables and fruits when you can find them. Lobby your greengrocer and supermarket to make more available. These foods contain the highest and best complement of minerals since the organic matter in the soil breaks down inorganic minerals (which your body can't use) and turns them into an organic form. *There is no way to compensate for the structural information missing when the organic matter in the soil has been destroyed by chemical farming.*

● Stress fresh vegetables above all else – they are highly complex and carry a high quality of structural information and order to feed your body. They are also rich in anti-cancer/anti-ageing compounds. Eat them either raw or lightly cooked at 2 meals a day.

● Unless you are vegetarian, eat organic meat and chicken. They not only taste better, but have a quite different fat content and come from much healthier animals who have themselves been fed on vegetable matter high in structural information and life order.

● Eat fresh fruit, preferably organic.

● Eat only whole grain cereals and breads, pasta and crackers, without added sugar or chemicals.

● Eat live yogurt, pure butter and naturally fermented cheeses as well as free-range eggs.

● Prepare as many of your foods as you can from scratch. Preparing a salad or some raw muesli for breakfast or a lovely country soup is a creative act. We use it as a kind of recreation. Teach others who live with you (especially children or a husband) to cook as well so the responsibility for meal preparation is shared. Then it remains a creative act and not a chore.

● Use extra virgin cold-pressed olive oil for cooking and salads.

● Eat 2 or 3 tablespoons of cold pressed flaxseed oil a day or 3-6 tablespoons of raw linseeds mixed into your breakfast yogurt or on your salad (see Resources, p.136). This is all you need to make sure you are getting the essential fatty acids in the cis form which your body requires for energy and long-lasting health.

● Eat 50-75% of your foods raw. Raw fruits and vegetables, organic raw seeds and nuts and grains soaked overnight to break down their hard-to-digest starches are the highest of all foods in structural information. When you are under stress, increase the percentage of raw foods you eat upwards closer to the 75% mark. It is an effective way of creating more energy and balance for yourself when you need it most.

● Grow as many of your own foods as you can yourself. Make 3 or 4 raised beds if you have room in your garden which you close-crop all year round with vegetables. You can grow salad stuff in between rose bushes if you have a small garden. If you have no garden, grow sprouted seeds and grains in your kitchen window or on the sill in the bedroom. They are cheap, easy to produce and lots of fun.

● Make space for the sacred acts of food preparation and eating in your life. They should be a time for celebration, enjoyment and relaxation. Learn to play again.

but beautifully packed meal with you – on the train, or on the plane. (Airline food is disgusting – an excellent example of just how dead food can become.) No matter where you eat or what time of day or night it is, give to every meal a feeling of improvisation and fun.

Cooking starts at the shopping stage. It is when you are in the market surrounded by great mounds of lettuces, avocados, fresh peppers, parsley and squid that you get your inspiration. Never set out to buy food with too fixed an idea of what you intend to buy. Look for what is particularly enticing. Some of the very best dishes can be made from the commonest, least expensive vegetables such as carrots, turnips and watercress and often the cheapest fish is the most tasty when prepared simply. While shopping you may come across something which, although you have not thought of it, is beautiful. It *draws* you to it. Buy it. Forget what you thought you were after. A good menu is created while you shop. Why seek something which is not there or out of season? Instead let yourself be tempted by what you find and make it the focus of your menu. Always *seek* temptation. To enjoy food fully, to celebrate the beauty of food, your senses need to be heightened. *Food should be so good that it feels sinful.*

Workbook *for* Energy grazing

Endless Energy food preparation breaks all the rules: throw out the convenience foods, put your kitchen scales away and leave aside all the complex routines you may have learned for preparing a good béchamel. Open wide your kitchen window to welcome the breezes of experiment, wit and spontaneity. In the realm of cooking a whole new ethos is born. Twenty years ago the most expensive and sought-after fabrics for clothes and decoration were synthetics, now cotton is at a premium. Just as our parents were fascinated with plastics and we go for natural woods and hand-woven baskets, so values in food preparation and eating have realigned themselves with natural resources. The traditional meal of beef Stroganoff with frozen vegetables smothered in hollandaise sauce, topped off with a piece of Black Forest Gateau, is replaced by something far more imaginative and hedonistic – slivers of wild Scottish salmon, two varieties of luscious garden-fresh salads, a slice or two of Russian black bread followed by a winter sorbet of cranberry and mint.

But in case you think you are *supposed* to eat lighter or more natural foods only because they will keep you from having a heart attack or prevent inches from creeping up around your waistline, think again. Yes, it's true *Endless Energy* cuisine will do all of these things. But the *real* joy of eating these fresh light foods lies in their taste, their texture and the remarkable ability they have to bring new life and excitement to a palate which has become jaded by too many highly processed, unimaginatively seasoned, overcooked dishes.

Endless Energy cooking reflects an attitude which is contemporary, joyous, pleasurable and hedonistic – a way of looking at life which *celebrates* the earth and its bounty and which not only takes from the planet what we need to nurture ourselves but also simultaneously nurtures the planet, by encouraging organic growing. Enjoy experimenting with it.

Grazing for energy

The way you eat does not change overnight – nor should it. If you want to create for yourself a high-energy way of eating, do it gradually. Look at the list below and tick any of the steps that are already part of your approach to eating. Then choose a new one to try. See if you can tick off one new step every week. By improving your diet bit by bit you are more likely to see your choices become permanent positive eating habits.

The 25 steps

1. Find healthy snack alternatives. See Snick Snacks and Snack Suggestions, p.96.
2. Replace icecream or puddings with live yogurt, combined with fruit and/or honey for a delicious dessert.
3. Buy yourself 2 or 3 packages of herb tea to try instead of tea or coffee (see Resources, p.137, for suggestions). Some teas are tasty iced. You can fill an empty mineral water bottle to drink chilled throughout the day.
4. If you aren't ready to give up coffee, try organic instead.
5. Wean yourself off sugar and sweeteners in tea or coffee. Instead,

use honey and decrease the amount gradually. As you re-educate your taste by eating fewer sweet foods, you will naturally want to eat less sugar in any form.

6. Don't skip breakfast.

7. Replace commercial breakfast cereals with Live Muesli, see recipe, p.95.

8. Become an avid label reader and shun anything containing artificial additives, preservatives, hydrogenated fats and sugars or artificial sweeteners. Check your cupboards, fridge or freezer for any of these items and make a mental note to find an alternative to them the next time you shop.

9. Before you tuck into a leg of deep-fried chicken or a cheeseburger make the mental connection that your body is made of what you put into it. Ask your body, not just your mind, if this is what you really want.

10. Make a commitment not to eat and run. Even if you are having a snack, eat it sitting down. Chew your foods well and allow your body a chance to digest them before you dash into a stressful activity.

11. Don't eat when you're emotionally upset or anxious, depressed or bored. Instead take a few minutes to write, exercise or meditate, or listen to some uplifting music.

12. Learn how to grow your own sprouts (see p.97).

13. Be *conscious* while you are eating and take time to enjoy the taste, texture and variety of your food.

14. Make 1 meal a day a glorious Master Salad (see p.94)

15. Find an organic source of meat, poultry and eggs.

16. Remove excess fat from meat before you cook it. Remove the skin from chicken.

17. Use skimmed milk instead of full-fat milk.

18. Drink filtered or bottled water instead of tap.

19. Learn to combine your foods well – particularly if you want to shed excess fat deposits (see p.97).

20. Try one or more of the natural energy enhancers such as spirulina (see p.101).

21. Try our Green Seasoning instead of table salt to flavour your foods (see p.95).

22. When you eat out in a restaurant, avoid items that have been cooked in fat. For instance, instead of fried fish in batter have grilled fish with lemon. Ask for sauces and salad dressings on the side so that you can leave them there if they are too rich or full of junk fats.

23. Vary your diet from day to day always looking for original new dishes to keep your taste buds happy.

24. Try the 5 Day Detox (p.65) to uncover hidden food sensitivities that may be depleting your energy levels or causing weight gain.

25. Treat yourself to an internal spring clean with the 7 day Cleanse (p.75).

The master salad

We feel about making salads the way the Japanese feel about tea ceremonies – salad-making is a sacred act, or it *should* be. Unfortunately what most people call a salad is a sad gathering of deceased vegetables. Yet, despite its unfortunate reputation, a good salad belongs to the realm of infinite culinary delights. We'd like to introduce you to the Master Salad so the thought (and the *taste*) of salad need never bore you again.

The secret of a Master Salad lies in the following 5 elements:

● **Use the best ingredients** Choose the freshest most flavourful vegetables you can find – ideally organically grown.

● **Go for imaginative combinations** Combine complementary flavours and textures for interest – use some ingredients raw and some cooked.

● **Get clever chopping:** Create variety by the way you chop, shred, dice or grate. (How you cut a vegetable actually makes a difference to how it tastes!)

● **Make irresistibly delicious dressings** A good dressing can make an indifferent salad great. A great dressing makes a great salad heaven!

● **Add tantalizing morsels** These give a salad its character and often provide not only interest but also substance in the form of protein.

The salad repertoire

The best salads are made from a combination of raw and cooked ingredients. Here are some suggestions.

The raw vegetable line-up

Leafy greens such as spinach, the lettuces – cos, Webb's Wonder, Chinese leaves, salad bowl, frissée, radicchio, lollo rosso, oak leaf, lamb's tongue – watercress, mustard and cress, red and white cabbage, carrots, beetroot, radishes, baby turnips, baby parsnips, celeriac, chicory, fennel, red, yellow and green sweet peppers, cauliflower, broccoli, avocados, spring onions, mangetout, baby peas, tomatoes, cucumber, courgettes, celery, mushrooms.

The cooked vegetables

- **Sautéed** The following vegetables are especially delicious wok-fried or sautéed in a heavy pan with olive oil before being added hot or cold to the salad: mushrooms, onion, shredded white or red cabbage, mangetout, french beans, courgettes, finely grated beetroot, peppers.
- **Steamed** Although they can also be enjoyed raw, broccoli and cauliflower are particularly nice lightly steamed in a salad. Steamed asparagus and french beans are also tasty.
- **Grilled** Aubergines, sweet peppers, courgettes and fennel sliced lengthwise and grilled with olive oil and garlic like the Italians do, develop a wonderful flavour.
- **Potato plus** Boiled or baked in their jackets and chopped into salads, potatoes give body and a contrasting soft texture.

Keep extra cooked salad goodies refrigerated in an airtight container to help make 'instant' salads.

Living proof

Home-grown organic sprouted seeds, cereals and pulses such as alfalfa, lentil, mung, chick pea, and fenugreek, sunflower seeds, wheat and barley bring pure vitality to a salad (see instructions on p.94).

Magic morsels

- **Hard-boiled eggs** Finely grated hard-boiled eggs add texture and body. They are especially delicious in spinach or lettuce-based salads.
- **Toasted seeds and nuts** Put sunflower, pumpkin or sesame seeds; almonds, cashews or hazelnuts into a frying pan and brown them until golden, stirring

to prevent them from burning. Add them to almost any salad combination for crunchiness.

- **Oven-roasted sprouts** Place 3-4 day wheat, barley or soya bean sprouts on a baking tray and sprinkle with sea salt or vegetable bouillon powder. Bake for 15 minutes in a moderate oven. They become crunchy and make delicious sweet salad croutons.
- **Super seaweeds** Soak or steam arame seaweed until tender, then add to salad. Marry the seaweed flavour with tamari and ginger in your dressing. Or toast Nori sheets over a hot plate until crispy and then crumble into a salad.
- **Tasty morsels from a tin** Keep the following tins handy to liven up a salad that 'lacks something': sweetcorn (without added sugar), hearts of palm, artichoke hearts, olives, capers, tuna fish (packed in brine), anchovies.

Use only the best

Choose your salad dressing ingredients from the very best available. The ultimate is cold-pressed olive oil. If you can get very fresh walnut or hazelnut oil they are also a real treat for dressings. Cold-pressed flaxseed oil makes an energy-enhancing addition.

- **Favourite vinegars** Cider, raspberry and umeboshi. The latter is made from fermented Japanese umeboshi plums and is fairly hard to find. It has a distinctive tangy flavour which is wonderful in dressings. Lemons or limes are also nice instead of vinegar in a vinaigrette dressing.
- **Tahini** (sesame seed paste) Can be used to make a Tahini Mayonnaise with water (see recipe, p.95)

and may be added to oil-based dressings to give a creamy texture and nutty flavour.

- **Tamari** (wheat-free soya sauce) adds richness to a dressing.
- **Worcestershire Sauce** There are also other tantalizing Lea & Perrins sauces such as Ginger and Orange and Chilli and Garlic. Although they contain a little sugar, these delicious sauces are quick and add flavour to dressings.
- **Sun-dried tomatoes, olive paste or pesto sauce** All of these come in a jar and add spice and originality to a dressing.
- **Mustards** We use whole grain Meaux mustard liberally in most of our dressings.
- **Fresh herbs and spices** Some can be grown in pots in your kitchen year-round, giving a refreshingly vivid flavour to salads. Some of our favourites include garlic, chives, coriander, basil, marjoram, parsley, thyme, lovage and fresh ginger root.
- **Fresh flower petals** These add appetizing colour. We like chive flower heads or marigold petals.
- **Vegetable bouillon powder** We use this bouillon powder in most of our dressings and many of our other dishes instead of salt. When we do use salt, our favourite variety is the tasty Maldon Salt Flakes.
- **Green Seasoning** This delicious, zesty powder is adapted from a recipe by Joyce Pearce – an inspiring friend of ours in New Zealand who cured herself of cancer with a high-raw diet. Add a teaspoon to salad dressing or sprinkle it onto a Master Salad, baked potato or bowl of soup (see recipe p.95).
- **Tofu** Although rather bland on its own, tofu can make a good base for dips or creamy dressings.

Energy recipes

The following recipes are designed to give you a taste of Endless Energy eating. You do not have to stick slavishly to the instructions we have given – they are only guidelines. If, for instance, a recipe calls for broccoli and you hate it, you can quite easily substitute cauliflower. The idea is to take the recipes and adapt them to *your* taste, making them your own. A note on quantity: most of the following recipes are designed to feed between 2-4 people. As the quantities are approximate (we both find measuring food cramps a cook's style), the amounts can easily be adjusted to suit your own particular needs.

Where measuring is important we have used the American measures as follows:
1C = one cup or eight fluid ounces (about the size of a large tea cup).
1T = one tablespoon
1t = one teaspoon.

Master salads

Set the scene by playing your favourite music, pour yourself a glass of juice, sparkling water or even organic wine, take a deep breath and enter the realm of the Master Salad.

First, choose a beautiful salad bowl. Our favourites are made of wood or glass. Sometimes, for visual appeal, we like to create a salad on a platter.

Gather your ingredients together and get creative. Here are some examples to inspire you:

Broccoli and hazelnuts

Tear a few leaves of salad bowl or Webb's Wonder lettuce into bite-sized pieces. Lightly steam several broccoli florets. Drain them and slice into bite-sized morsels. Toast a handful of hazelnuts in a frying pan until golden. Peel and dice an avocado. (If the avocado is thick skinned it's easiest to halve it, remove the stone and slice it horizontally and vertically within the skin, then scoop out the diced flesh with a spoon.) Halve several cherry tomatoes. Place all the ingredients in a salad bowl together with a handful of alfalfa or mixed sprouts and a few leaves of fresh basil. Toss with Spicy Vinaigrette dressing and serve. If the cooked ingredients are still warm, so much the better!

Crunchy potato salad

Potatoes make a comforting and filling salad – especially welcome on gloomy winter days. Coarsely grate 1-2 carrots. Chop 2 sticks of celery lengthwise and then across into small pieces. (In general the smaller you chop vegetables the more flavour they have.) Dice half a red pepper. Chop 2 potatoes in their jackets. Mix the ingredients together with a handful of wheat sprouts and some freshly chopped parsley. Serve with Tahini Mayonnaise.

Spicy oriental salad

This salad demands to be eaten with chopsticks. It is an ideal introduction to seaweed for the wary. Soak half a packet of arame seaweed for 20 minutes or until tender and drain. Chop 1 or 2 carrots into matchsticks – cutting first crossways on a diagonal and then slicing these ovals lengthways into sticks. Chop a bunch of watercress crossways into bite-sized pieces. Finely shred 2-3 slices of red cabbage. Slice 1-2 courgettes crossways and fry in a pan with olive oil until golden. Toast a handful of pumpkin or sesame seeds until they 'pop'. Combine all the ingredients and toss with a vinaigrette dressing to which you add 1-2 teaspoons of finely grated fresh ginger root and some finely chopped chives.

Smooth spinach salad

Made with tender young organic spinach this salad is sheer delight. Tear several spinach leaves into bite-sized pieces. Halve a few radishes. Finely dice $^{1}/_{2}$ a head of fennel. Finely chop a ripe tomato. Slice several tinned hearts of palm crossways. Dice an avocado. Finely grate 1-2 hard-boiled eggs. Combine all the ingredients in a bowl with a few pitted black olives and toss with a garlic-flavoured vinaigrette dressing.

Irresistible dressings
Spicy vinaigrette

We use this vinaigrette, or one of its variations, more than any other dressing. Place the following ingredients in the bottom of a screw top jar: 2t of wholegrain mustard, 1t vegetable bouillon powder, the juice of one lemon or 4T of cider vinegar, 1t of tamari. Then add one or more of the following: 1T chopped fresh herbs such as basil, marjoram and parsley; or 1t of finely grated ginger root; or 1 clove of garlic (pressed); or 1t (heaped) of sun-dried tomatoes or olive paste or pesto sauce; season to taste with freshly ground pepper and Green Seasoning (optional – see recipe on this page) to taste. Add 1C of cold-pressed olive oil and shake to combine the ingredients.

Tahini mayonnaise

A tasty and healthy substitute for conventional mayonnaise – good with tuna or slaw-type salads. Combine the following ingredients in a food processor or blender: ½C tahini, the juice of a large lemon and a teaspoon of grated lemon rind, 1T of finely chopped onion (optional), 1t of French mustard, ½C of water, 1t of vegetable bouillon powder. Blend in the food processor or blender until the Tahini Mayonnaise is smooth.

Creamy tofu

You can serve this creamy dressing as a filling for baked potatoes or use it as a dip with crudités. Combine the following in a blender or food processor: 10oz tofu, 1 heaped teaspoon of mustard, the juice of 1 lemon, 1-2t umeboshi vinegar or tamari, 1-2t freshly grated ginger root, a few fresh or dried herbs such as coriander or thyme and marjoram. Blend well and serve.

Curried avocado

This dressing is so delicious you'll want to eat it from the spoon! Combine the following ingredients in a food processor: the flesh of 1-2 ripe avocados, 1C of fresh squeezed orange juice, 1t curry powder, 2t vegetable bouillon

powder, a few lovage leaves or some fresh parsley and 1 clove of garlic (optional). Blend until smooth. For a stiff dip, add slightly less juice, for a thinner dressing, use slightly more.

Green seasoning powder

A wonderful addition to dressings. Take 4T kelp powder, 1T vegetable bouillon powder, 1t curry powder, 1t celery seeds (ground), 1t fresh grated ginger root, 4 cloves garlic. Blend all of the above ingredients in a food processor, adding the garlic last. Place on a plate or flat dish and leave to dry in a warm place for 1-2 hours (the top of an Aga or radiator is ideal). Pour into a salt cellar and use to flavour your food at the table or in recipes.

LIVE MUESLI

One of the tastiest breakfasts we know. This recipe is similar to the original muesli developed by the famous Swiss physician Max Bircher-Benner. Unlike store-bought dried muesli which can sit heavily in your stomach, this one is made with fresh fruit and soaked grains which are easy to digest and leave you feeling satisfied and light.

1-2T oat flakes (you can also use millet, barley or rye flakes) soaked overnight in a little water or fruit juice to help break down the starch into sugars, a handful of raisins (soaked with the oats), 1 apple or firm pear (grated), 1 small banana (finely chopped), a squeeze of fresh lemon juice, 2T plain yogurt (optional), 1t honey (optional), 1T chopped nuts such as almonds, brazils or hazels, 1T powdered cinnamon.

Combine the oat flakes and raisins with the grated apple/pear and banana and add a squeeze of lemon juice. Top with a little yogurt, then drizzle with honey, sprinkle with ground nuts and cinnamon, and savour.

You can vary live muesli dozens of ways by using different types of fresh fruit such as pineapple, peaches or berries, depending on what's available. You can also soak different dried fruit, such as apricots, dates, sultanas, figs and pears when the range of fresh fruits available is limited. For other delicious breakfast ideas see the suggestions in the 7 Day Cleanse Diet p.75.

Wok-fried vegetables

You can use almost any combination of vegetables in this recipe. It is a lovely way to eat salad warm. Take a handful of cashew nuts (or other nuts/seeds), 1 onion sliced into rings, 1 diced red pepper, a few mushrooms, some cauliflower florets, a few mangetout (topped and tailed), 1 courgette cut into slices, a handful of sprout mix, some tamari sauce and olive oil.

Heat a wok or frying pan and add a thin layer of olive oil. Toss in the cashew nuts and cook until golden. Add the vegetables, beginning with the onions and the cauliflower florets which take longest to cook. After a couple of minutes add the courgette, mangetout, red pepper and sprouts. Fry until they are cooked, but still lightly crunchy. Season with tamari and serve.

Souper soups

We eat this type of soup often – especially in the winter. You can vary the recipe endless ways to suit your taste. Two particularly delicious additions are chicken and barley.

Hearty vegetable soup

1 large onion, 2 leeks, 3 sticks of celery, 1-2 carrots, 1 turnip, 1 parsnip, 2 medium-sized potatoes, 1C fresh garden peas or lentil sprouts, 2T olive oil, 1 litre of boiling water, 1T bouillon powder, 1-2t Herbes de Provence.

Wash and scrub the vegetables. Peel the onion. Dice the root vegetables and celery into small cubes and finely chop the onion and leek. Sauté the leek and onion in the olive oil in a large cooking pot. Add the celery, carrots, turnip, parsnip and potatoes and put on the lid. Allow the vegetables to sweat for 5 minutes. Add the boiling water, bouillon powder and herbs and simmer for 30-40 minutes. Add the peas (or sprouts) and cook for a further 15 minutes.

Instant soup

This is our answer to the TV dinner. It is ideal when you want a quick light supper.

1t vegetable bouillon powder, an egg, a spring onion (finely chopped) and a squeeze of fresh garlic, a sheet of toasted Nori seaweed or a few toasted sesame seeds, a drop or two of Tabasco sauce or a little tamari, and boiling water.

Stir the bouillon powder into a mug of boiling water. Whisk an egg into the broth with a fork (it will 'cook' almost instantly). Add the garlic and the spring onion. Sprinkle crumbled Nori and/or a few toasted sesame seeds on top. Season with Tabasco or tamari. Drink with the help of a spoon.

Snick snacks

If you're looking for an alternative to chocolate bars or biscuits to snack on, try this delicious recipe. The Snick Snacks combine a quick energy source, in simple fruit sugars, together with sustained energy from nuts and seeds to tide you over between meals.

$1/2$C almonds, $1/4$C sunflower seeds, $1/2$C dried dates, $1/2$C dried figs, 2T desiccated coconut, $1/2$t natural vanilla essence, 1T malt extract (available from health food stores) or honey, carob powder (optional).

Toast the almonds and sunflower seeds in a frying pan and then grind coarsely in a food processor. Add the dried dates and figs and blend until well combined. Put the mixture in a bowl and stir in the coconut, vanilla essence and malt extract or honey. Form into little balls with your hands and roll in carob powder. Refrigerate and enjoy between meals with a cup of herb tea. For a variation, replace the coconut with 2T of spirulina powder and 2T whole raisins for their chewy texture. The spirulina powder is excellent addition as it helps satisfy hunger pangs.

Other snack suggestions

- Toasted sunflower seeds and pumpkin seeds.
- Homemade popcorn with a little sea salt or Green Seasoning (p.95).
- Carob Pods (sometimes called St John's Bread) – the dried pods can be chewed in place of a chocolate bar.
- Apples.
- Crudités such as carrot, celery and red pepper sticks. Also good for a packed lunch together with a delicious dip (see recipes, p.95).
- Oatcakes (sugar-free) or rice cakes (both available from health food shops). Enjoy them plain with your tea or juice, or spread with a little butter or nutbutter.
- Fresh squeezed vegetable juice (keep in a flask with ice cubes to protect from oxidation).
- Hot spicy apple juice – put concentrated apple juice (available from a health-food shop) in a mug and add boiling water and allspice or cinnamon to taste.

Wonder sprouts

We cannot recommend sprouts highly enough. Not only can they be grown in your kitchen to provide delicious and inexpensive organic salads all year round, but they boast some extraordinary energy-giving properties. When a seed, pulse or grain begins to germinate it becomes a wondrous energy factory producing vast amounts of essential nutrients. For instance, the vitamin E content of wheat grains – already one of the best sources in nature – increases up to 3 times upon sprouting. The B2 content of oats rises by at least 1300 per cent. Apart from the vitamins, sprouts also contain considerable quantities of minerals and even protein, all in readily assimilable form. The process of germination, like the process of digestion, converts complex energy reserves into the simple energy compounds needed for metabolism. Sprouts are in effect a 'pre-digested' food, so that when you eat them your body is able to absorb their nourishment. They are also rich in chlorophyll which supports your body's production of haemoglobin (the oxygen-carrying molecule in the blood), vital for cell energy metabolism.

In just a few minutes a day you can cultivate a continual sprout supply so that you never run out of fresh salad ingredients. One of the simplest ways to grow a variety of sprouts is as a mix. We particularly like a combination of alfalfa with lentil and mung. To this we occasionally add a few fenugreek or radish seeds for extra zest. Another of our favourites are wheat sprouts which have a delicious chewy texture and nutty flavour. These we sprout on their own because they are ready so quickly – usually in 2-3 days. Incidentally, even someone with a food sensitivity to wheat can usually enjoy wheat sprouts problem-free, thanks to the changes that occur in the grain during germination.

Below are instructions on how to grow our sprout mix. Once you get hooked on growing your own sprouts you might like to try some of the more exotic ones. (See Further Reading, p.140, for a good book on sprouting/sprout recipes.)

DIY sprout mix

In a large glass jar place 6T of alfalfa seeds and 2T each of lentils and mung beans. Fill the jar with water and leave to soak for about 12 hours (or overnight). Drain the excess water away by placing a sieve over the neck of the jar, and then rinse and drain twice more. Divide the mixture between two (or more) jars so that there are no more than two inches of sprouts in each. This way your sprouts will have sufficient room to breathe and grow. Rinse and drain the sprouts twice a day.

Alternatively take a seed tray and line it with paper kitchen towels, then spread the sprout mix over the bottom of it. Simply spray the sprouts with water from a plant spray twice a day and stir them around gently for aeration. After 4-6 days, when the alfalfa seeds have developed little green leaves, the mix is ready to harvest. Rinse the sprouts well and drain. Store them in the fridge in an air-tight container or in sealed polythene bags to be used abundantly in salads and other vegetable dishes.

Sprout burgers

1C of almonds or a mixture of almonds with sunflower seeds, 1-2C wheat sprouts, 2 carrots, 2-3 spring onions, 1 egg, 1 clove garlic, 2t vegetable bouillon, dash of Worcestershire sauce, fresh parsley (finely chopped), olive oil.

Grind the almonds (or almonds and sunflower seeds) in the food processor and place in a bowl. Blend the wheat sprouts until fairly gooey and add to the nuts. Finely grate the carrots and chop the spring onions. Stir the ingredients together and add the seasonings. Finally stir an egg into the mixture to help bind it. Form the mix into patties with your hands and fry in olive oil. Sprinkle with fresh parsley and serve. Makes about 12-16 vegetarian burgers.

Right-on combinations

One of the golden rules of eating for energy is Don't Mix Foods That Fight. Strange as it may seem, some of the most popular dishes in our culture, such as fish and chips, spaghetti bolognese, or roast beef and potatoes, actually provoke mini stomach battles. Here's why.

The human body functions at its best when only one form of concentrated food is eaten at a time. A concentrated food is anything that is not a fruit or a vegetable capable of being eaten raw. They fall into 2 categories: concentrated proteins, such as fish, steak, shellfish, eggs, yogurt, nuts; and concentrated starches which include bread, pasta, grains, beans and potatoes. Concentrated proteins require an acid medium to be properly digested. Concentrated starches need an alkaline one. When you eat a meal that includes both, neither the starches nor the proteins have their ideal pH medium. Digestion is slowed down and can be incomplete. This can lead to digestive upsets and feelings of hunger or cravings. It also encourages a build up of toxicity in the system.

Apart from separating concentrated starches and proteins, it's also important to eat fruit away from other foods. The reason is that fruit is digested incredibly quickly, sometimes remaining in the stomach for as little as 15-20 minutes. If you eat fruit at a meal with other foods it may be forced to remain in the stomach for 2 or more hours. During this time the fruit can start to ferment, resulting in indigestion and wind. If you want to eat fruit with a meal it is best to have it as a starter and leave 20 minutes before the next course.

So what foods *can* you eat together? Basically most raw or cooked vegetables are digested quite happily along with either a concentrated protein (fish, eggs, nuts) or a concentrated starch (baked potatoes, rice, lentils). Because of their digestibility, we consider sprouted grains, pulses and seeds as 'vegetables'. Strict food combiners separate fruits into 3 categories: acid, sub-acid and sweet, and insist that these should be eaten separately. We have found that as long as we eat fruit on its own, we can combine different varieties without any difficulty.

Food combining is not something to become neurotic or anxious about. Some people with strong digestive systems seem to be able to mix anything together and come out feeling full of energy. Nevertheless for anyone who tends to suffer from indigestion or a weight problem, wise combining can be a real blessing.

The powerhouses

When it comes to nutritional supplements, we both prefer to use complexes from nature rather than collections of vitamins and minerals. Sometimes we make an exception and use a specific vitamin or mineral in a highly bio-available form – like chromium polynictinate for instance or vitamin C. But we find that many natural complexes work far better than artificially produced vitamins and inorganic forms of minerals. (In fact, almost all vitamins are artificially made for there is no

other way of producing them.) Here are some of the supplements we like best and use often.

Perfect probiotics

There is a lot of talk about acidophilus and how good it is for maintaining a healthy colony of intestinal flora. The healthy human gastrointestinal tract plays host to a huge and varied population of micro organisms – so much so that an amazing 30% of the weight of a stool is made up by bacteria. When you take antibiotics, the drugs not only kill off whatever *destructive* bacteria they have been taken for, they can also wipe out your natural colony of *beneficial* micro organisms which are there to help protect your body from infection, to produce important B-Complex vitamins, to detoxify your system and to keep the acid/alkaline balance of your intestines in good balance. If this helpful colony of micro organisms becomes depleted as a result of antibiotics, poor eating or stress then undesirable 'beasties' such as E coli, Staphylococci, s. aureus, and yeasts such as Candida albicans can replace them to undermine your health, deplete your energy and unbalance your body's biochemistry.

It can be helpful to supplement your diet with a good probiotic – a product that supports the growth of helpful micro organisms in the gut. The problem is, as a big independent study recently showed, most probiotics and lactobacillus acidophilus products are useless. Their micro organism count is either too low or not skilfully protected and they are broken down and destroyed in the stomach before they ever reach the

colon. Choose a lactobacillus acidophilus and Bifido bacterium product which is milk-free, supplies at least 1 billion organisms per capsule, is taken from human strains, is stabilized and has a good shelf life. Such a product is almost a necessity when eliminating Candida albicans. Anything less will be a waste of your money.

Enzyme helpers

Digestive enzymes such as amylase, protease, lipase and bromelin are essential to break down the foods you eat into usable nutrients. The healthy body produces its own enzymes each of which has a specific job to do, like break down fats or break down proteins or cellulose in the foods you eat. Crash dieting, chlorine in drinking water, poor eating, stress or deficiencies of specific minerals or vitamins needed for your body to produce these enzymes, can mean your enzyme supply is depleted so you are unable to break your foods down properly. (Ageing can also be a reason for this.) The result can be food sensitivities with all of the troublesome physical and emotional problems they cause, or indigestion, or a lowering of energy after you have eaten, or the kind of digestive disturbance that causes feelings of hunger after a meal and triggers overeating.

Like good probiotics, a good digestive enzyme product can be hard to find. There is one exceptional one. It is based on enzymes of plant origins which are biologically active and able to maintain their activity over a wide range of pH changes in the body. Unlike animal-derived enzymes which frequently turn rancid, these vegetable-based ones are high potency and very stable. One with each meal can make a remarkable difference to many people with enzyme deficiencies (see Resources, p.136).

Oil power for energy

The kind of oils and fats you use matter a great deal if you want to live your own brand of endless energy. Oils and fats come in three forms: saturated – butter and animal fats which have a very low activity of electron transfer; mono-unsaturate – *extra virgin* olive oils for instance, which are moderately active and also relatively stable, therefore good to use when cooking; and poly-unsaturated – corn oil, groundnut oil, sunflower oil and safflower which have 2 or more double bonds and are highly active as well as highly unstable and prone to rancidity. Use butter on your breads and potatoes. Use olive oil for wok-frying foods. For your salad dressings use olive oil ideally mixed 50/50 with pure cold-pressed flaxseed oil.

Flaxseed oil is the best polyun-saturated oil you can find for supplying essential fatty acids in your diet. It is a superb combination of both omega 3 and omega 6 essential fatty acids in excellent balance. It, too, is highly unstable but also highly active – to encourage energy transfer. And it is hard to come by. It must be bought fresh and under refrigeration, then kept refrigerated once opened and used within weeks or it goes rancid. Fresh flaxseed oil taken either in capsules or mixed with extra virgin olive oil on your salads has been shown to clear up cases of pre-menstrual syndrome, asthma, allergies, water retention in women, skin conditions and also to enhance vitality – all within a month. But it doesn't work unless the flax seed oil is of the highest quality and absolutely fresh (see Resources, p.136).

Other good sources of essential fatty acids include fresh fish such as mackerel, herring, sardines, anchovies, and wild trout. All are good sources of the right kind of natural polyunsaturated oils. Salmon is too but *farmed* salmon is not. Because of the diet on which the salmon are fed the levels of essential fatty acids are significantly lower in cultured fish than in wild fish.

Bones, nails and hair

Bones, nails and hair have one thing in common: in order to stay healthy and strong they need plenty of minerals.

Their strength builds up to a maximum density by the age of 35. After that, provided you eat well and get plenty of regular aerobic exercise, the bone strength you develop in your 30s lasts a lifetime. There is a lot of nonsense talked about calcium supplements and the prevention of osteoporosis. First of all, calcium alone doesn't work to build strong bones and nails and hair. It never did. For it to be absorbed, you need optimal quantities of zinc, copper, boron, manganese, magnesium and vitamin D in your diet and – in many ways most important of all – silica. Secondly, most of the calcium pills on the market are pretty useless. To give you some idea: in a 1000mg pill of calcium gluconate (the most common form) you will find only 90mg of calcium. To get the recommended amount of calcium for a woman each day you would have to take about 15 of these horse tablets. Better to get plenty of exercise and take a really good supplement of 500-600mg of highly bio-available calcium plus one of magnesium, as well as the same quantity of organic silica, which has the remarkable ability to bind all of these precious minerals into hard tissues such as nails and bones and hair (see Resources, p.136).

Out with hot flushes

One of the more annoying energy changes in women is the experience of hot flushes before menstruation or at the menopause. The standard medical advice to menopausal women is to take Hormone Replacement Therapy (HRT). We wouldn't touch it with a 10 foot pole. This is first because, given the delicate balance in the body that exists between the various endocrine glands such as the pituitary, ovaries, adrenals and thyroid, there is no way in which you can give one specific hormone without unbalancing the works. Secondly, since a woman's endocrine system is the interface between spirit and body, to do so can interfere profoundly with her spiritual development and her capacity to move on to the next stage of her life. Menopause itself is a watershed, a time of profound change. Once a woman comes to terms with this change, it can also be her greatest gateway to personal freedom and creativity. She is open to new energies, she breaks through the barriers of expectation that until then have bound her into the roles of mother, wife and *conventional* woman. Taking hormones such as oestrogen and progesterone can strongly interfere with this passage to freedom and lock her artificially into child-bearing mode which she is ready at this time in her life to leave behind.

How do you deal with hot flushes if they come? And with the feelings of profound uncertainty that happen whenever there is such deep change taking place? First by honouring your core energy so that the 'fire' that covers your body in the midst of a hot flush becomes transmuted into the fires of creation out of which your new life is to be made. Secondly by transforming your diet into one that supports health at the very highest levels, and by reclaiming your body through conscious awareness and physical activity. Cut out every form of highly processed food including all junk fats from your diet. Consider adding nutritional supplements such as pure cold-pressed flaxseed oil (see p.99), as well as calcium EAP, magnesium EAP, organic silica and finally Vitamin E and the bioflavonoids. Oestrogen in a woman's body competes with the bioflavonoids to maintain the integrity of capillaries. There is a close similarity between some bioflavonoids and a female hormone etradiol diethye-stilbestrol. During menopause and just before a period, when there is a big drop in oestrogen levels in a woman's body, the epithelium of the capillaries become thinner, more fragile and ready to leak. It is then that hot flushes take place. An excellent double blind study carried out at Loyola University using vitamin C and bioflavonoids showed that 6 tablets a day (each containing 150mg of hesperidin complex, 50mg of hesperidin methyl chalcone and 200 mg vitamin C) helped most of the women gain relief. We have suggested supplements of the bioflavonoids, vitamin C and 100-250 mg of vitamin E to be taken daily to many women with this complaint, and have had good feedback from the women who have tried it.

Bee powerful

There is nothing like bee products to support high-level energy and wellbeing – especially propolis. This sticky resinous substance exuded by the leaf buds and bark of trees which is gathered by bees to cement their hives is a superb natural antibiotic. In capsules of 200-250mg it helps keep the digestive system clean and free of thrush, relieves cold and 'flu symptoms as well as energizing the body as a whole. It comes in tincture form for internal and external use. We find it helpful for sore throats, gum problems and as a gargle. You can even put it on warts and verrucas. It also comes, mixed with honey, as a mouth-wash and an excellent toothpaste with antiseptic properties. Propolis is rich in flavonoids so it can also be useful in women who get hot flushes before a period or at the menopause. The trouble is a lot of propolis, like pure bee pollen (which we also use in small quantities for its protein, mineral and B-vitamin content), is not pure because it comes from areas where the bees have been sugar fed or where they draw nectar from flowers that have been sprayed with pesticides. We prefer the purest propolis, honeys and pollens, many of which are organically produced in areas of New Zealand (see Resources, p.137).

Amazon power

The most exciting herb we have come across for a long time is Suma (Pfaffia paniculata). Locally known as Para Todo ('for everything'), Suma has been used by Brazilian Indians for centuries as an aphrodisiac and tonic. Recent research has discovered that, like pure ginseng (which is almost impossible to find and prohibitively expensive when you do), the wild root of the Suma plant has powerful adaptogenic properties.

The adaptogens have been well studied by the Russian scientists who first coined the word. They are substances which, in carefully conducted laboratory and clinical studies, have been shown to enhance an organism's 'non-specific resistance' to ageing, illness and fatigue. In practical terms an adaptogen enhances your body's ability to adapt itself to all forms of stress – from fatigue, illness, exertion and ageing to the stress of emotional hardship – while at the same time normalizing biochemical activities. Adaptogens are often called 'medicines for well people'. They appear to have positive effects on the endocrine system helping to balance hormones naturally. They seem to be particularly helpful for the adrenal glands which support the body under stress. As such they can be enormously helpful in keeping young and full of vitality.

Amongst other constituents, Suma is rich in the saponins, some of which show anti-tumour activity and in a plant hormone called *ecdysone*. At the University of Sao Paulo, Dr Milton Brazzach, Chairman of Pharmacology, has treated thousands of patients with serious ailments including both diabetes and cancer and verified the plant's potent healing and preventative powers. Researchers have found that a major source of the plant's energy-enhancing and protective properties lie in its ability to detoxify connective tissue of what are called *homotoxins*. These are wastes which are not only locked into the tissues of cellulite in a woman's body but which also interfere with the active transport of nutrients to the cells and in the production of cellular energy, and lead long term to changes in the DNA associated with premature ageing and the development of degenerative diseases. What all of this means to the active woman is that Suma is well worth looking at as a nutritional support to raising your energy levels, enhancing your ability to be very active both mentally and physically without fatigue or damage, and detoxifying your cells as a prevention against premature ageing, cellulite and degeneration.

Green miracle of nature

An almost microscopic plant, spirulina is a form of fresh water algae which grows wild in Lake Chad in the Sahara where it has for generations been used as a natural source of protein. Taken in the form of powder mixed with vegetable or fruit juice or drunk hot in vegetable broth, spirulina is a unique nutritional supplement which offers the body a high degree of structural information in a form that is quickly and readily absorbed. It is probably nature's richest food source for minerals and vitamins and essential amino acids all wrapped up in a wonderful green synergy. 2 or 3 tablespoons a day help replenish many of the minerals needed after having lived on a diet of convenience foods for too long. Spirulina offers an excellent balance of essential amino acids in an alkaline form which are quickly and easily absorbed even by people with digestive difficulties. Taken 30 minutes before a meal it also curbs an overactive appetite. In a cup of broth it also makes an excellent meal-replacement when in a hurry. It is nature's richest food source of Vitamin B12, chelated organic iron, beta carotene, the anti-oxidant shown to have anti-cancer properties and probably also nature's richest source of other anti-oxidants as a group including Vitamin C, B1, B5, and B6 as well as zinc, manganese, Vitamin E and selenium. If we had to choose only one powerhouse from nature it would be spirulina. But beware. Not all spirulina on the market has been grown in clean water. Choose only the best in tablet or powder form (see Resources, p.137).

Chapter 10

Energy *in* motion

Nothing connects a woman with her own power so well as regular physical activity. It brings you in touch with your own body so you experience it as a living breathing organism capable of radical transformation rather than as an object separated from your *self* to be measured against media ideals and found wanting. Regular physical activity helps you to get to know yourself at the deepest levels and accept yourself wholeheartedly not only physically but in all your emotional and personal eccentricities as well. Finally, exercise carried out with a real awareness of being *in* your body, helps to heal splits between mind and body more easily than anything else.

Electrons in motion

The standard advice about exercise is that you should get plenty of it because it is good for you. All perfectly true. Regular aerobic exercise lowers cholesterol, enhances VO2Max (the measure of how well your body uses oxygen), gets rid of high blood pressure, protects you from premature ageing, and keeps sex hormone levels high. But this is only the beginning of what exercise has to offer.

In a living human body, movement breeds energy. Your body is a mass of atoms and molecules in constant motion. Their shifting and whirling creates clouds of electrons and organized masses of magnetic fields, starting at a sub-molecular level and going right on up to the level of your organs and glands and systems. An alive body – a body able to call on endless energy for thinking and feeling, movement and creativity – is a body in which heightened levels of electron transfer are commonplace and in which energies are highly ordered. Exercise helps you get your body that way and keep it that way.

Remember that law of physics which states that the passing of fluids through magnetic fields produces electromotive power? Aerobic exercise sets in motion the flow of liquids such as blood and lymph through magnetic fields of your body producing an abundance of internal magnetic energy. Aerobic exercise, where your heart is beating firmly and strongly and your breathing is deep, heightens fluid movement. It also puts a positive form of stress on your skeleton so that your bones produce electromagnetic energy every time you flex your muscles as well. Even the extra oxygen you take in while you move enlivens your cells, enhancing metabolic energy.

The physical, mental and spiritual rewards of exercise are so far-reaching that to say you *should* exercise because it lowers your cholesterol or firms your thighs sounds banal . It could better be said that the right kind of regular exercise can transform your life.

Mind blowing

Since the time of the ancient Greeks, physical exertion has been associated with an enhanced state of mind. This means a state of mind which includes feeling good, being free from anxiety, having a better quality of life and maintaining a healthy sense of detachment about what goes on from day to day, as well as having a strong sense of self-worth. The big irony is that the people who have the greatest need for exercise (as a result of carrying too much fat on their bodies, or because of a negative self-image) are often the least likely to exercise on their own initiative. This is particularly true of women for whom exercise, at least until the last decade or so, was considered unfeminine. Even now women are commonly inhibited by a number of things. First, low energy or depression which mean you lack the incentive to get physical and which can lead to a feeling of futility. Secondly, poor self-esteem and a feeling of helplessness – the sense that nothing you can do will make any difference. Thirdly, a feeling of being trapped in a body (particularly a flabby or overweight body) that you don't like coupled with an inability to imagine it ever changing. If you are willing to give exercise a real try, within six to twelve weeks all of these energy-blocking attitudes can be transformed.

Make depression a thing of the past

Clinical depression has certain characteristics: fatigue, low self-esteem, sadness, hopelessness, despair, pessimism and a sense of something (often youth or good looks) having been lost. Depression is predominantly a female experience. Statistics show that women suffer it six times more frequently than men. When this information first came out it provoked much discussion as to why. Is depression hormonally dependent? Is it a function of women often being relegated to second class citizens in our male intellectually dominated society? Does the lowered status in women create a sense of disempowerment and lead to a desire for approval which is seldom forthcoming? Probably there is some truth in all of these.

Many studies on the effect of aerobic exercise, such as brisk walking for 30 to 45 minutes a day or running, or swimming, or rebounding or rowing, have shown that putting sedentary people into an exercise programme significantly diminishes depression and all its associated characteristics. Exercise does this far better than anti-depressant medication (which is dangerous stuff anyway), psychotherapy or other standard treatments for depression.

Just how regular exercise banishes depression has caused a lot of speculation. One doctor, who is an expert in the field, suggests that the enhanced blood flow and oxygen to the tissues all over the body, when you exercise regularly, may influence the central nervous system and cause mood changes. Others suggest that since the brain hormone noradrenaline is known to be low in people who are depressed and since regular exercise raises it, this may be the cause. Whatever the hypothesis, what matters most is that regular exercise supports the wellbeing of bodymind *as a whole* superbly well. In doing so, it helps re-establish energetic harmony in every way.

Dissolving anxiety

Like depression, chronic anxiety can also cripple your spirit and wreak havoc with your body. It is another experience particularly common among women. It wastes volumes of energy that could otherwise be expressed in joy and creativity. When you are anxious, you worry, you can't concentrate properly and you frequently have trouble relaxing or sleeping. Chronic anxiety can also result in unpleasant physical symptoms such as muscle tension, nausea, hot sweats and a high pulse rate. Studies carried out to determine the effects of regular aerobic exercise on anxiety have turned up interesting results. Exercise can be used to lift anxiety and restore peacefulness and mental clarity but, to do this, the exercise must be *low-intensity*. Work out too hard and it will only make your anxiety worse.

Easy does it

We in the West have this weird notion that if a little of something does you good, twice as much good will come from a double dose. When it comes to physical activity as part of an endless-energy lifestyle (as opposed to busting a gut to win a medal at the next Olympics), nothing could be further from the truth. It is low-intensity exercise which is transformative, not pushing yourself to your limits or going for the burn. This means exercising at around seventy per cent of your maximum heart rate (MHR) for 30 to 45 minutes between three and six times a week – not harder (see Your Maximum Heart Rate). It is the same kind of exercise which can be used to exchange body fat for beautifully toned muscles.

Fat is your body's way of storing fuel. How rapidly this fuel gets used up depends upon your basic metabolic rate. One of the reasons fat people hold on to their fat is that their metabolic rate is sluggish. (Crash dieting, by the way, lowers your metabolic rate even further so you get fat on less and less food.) A lot of the prescription diet pills on the market with nasty side effects work by temporarily speeding up your metabolic rate in an unhealthy way. Exercise does it safely in a way that, so long as you keep up your physical activities, is *permanent*.

Go for the smoulder

For physical activity to burn body fat and exchange it for muscle the exercise you do has to be regular, consistent, rhythmic and to involve large muscle groups. It also has to be carried out within your ideal target range – that is at about seventy to eighty-five per cent of your MHR. Whatever aerobic activity you choose, you need to bring your heart rate within that range and keep it there for the duration of the session.

There is a lot of irrelevant information given about how many calories you burn during different activities. The implication is that the harder you work out (that is the closer you are to the eighty-five per cent MHR figure), the more fat you will lose. So a lot of women start running or swimming, push themselves extra

---

YOUR MAXIMUM HEART RATE

Your target rate for physical activity is 70-85% of your maximum heart rate. Here is how to calculate your own MHR:

Subtract your age from 220. For instance if you are 36 years old, your MHR would be 220 minus 36 or 184. Your ideal aerobic range is then figured by multiplying that number by 0.7 for the low end and 0.85 for the high. For this 36 year old that works out at 129 to 156 beats per minute. When you are exercising within this range it is considered safe. If you are exercising to help raise your self-esteem, get rid of depression and anxiety or encourage fat loss from your body, you need to exercise so your heart rate stays around the lower figure – 129.

Here's how to take your pulse during exercise:
After a few minutes of exercising, stop and put 3 fingers over the radial artery at your wrist to find your heart beat. Using a watch with a second hand count the number of heart beats over a period of 15 seconds. Then multiply this by 4 and you will know immediately if you are working out in the right range.

---

hard, get exhausted, wonder why it isn't working, get discouraged and give up. The truth is that at the higher end of your target rate your body will take more of its fuel from the glycogen in your muscles, burning sugar instead of fat. Your body burns fat well only in the lower target range, around seventy per cent of MHR. This means that you can exercise more easily, stay at it longer, not experience the mental fatigue that comes with using up glycogen stores and, at the same time, offer your body maximum support for fat burning.

Regular exercise also helps maintain the proper levels of growth hormone in your body. Growth hormone declines with age, probably more as a result of biochemical and energetic imbalances in the body (*certainly* as a result of inactivity) than the passing of the years themselves. When growth hormone levels are up, your body builds muscle. When they fall, you lay down fat. Going on and off crash diets in an attempt to lose weight interferes with growth hormone production and encourages your body to replace muscle tissue with fat.

Fat burning for energy

Co-Enzyme Q10 (COQ), taken as a nutritional supplement on an empty stomach, can be enormously helpful both in encouraging energy release from fat deposits via the mitochondria – your cells' 'furnaces' where fat is burnt – and in fuelling muscle activity while you are exercising. It can increase your endurance, enhance immunity, and it acts as an anti-oxidant helping to prevent free-radical damage. COQ plays a crucial role in ATP energy production by facilitating electron transfer thanks to its propensity to donate electrons and release energy for body use. Studies show that COQ supplements significantly increase exercise tolerances and improve electrocardiograms during treadmill testing. Athletes who use COQ to improve performance and as part of an anti-ageing regime take 30-60mg a day.

Chromium muscles

Few people in the West get enough chromium in their diets because food refining removes much of it and our high consumption of refined sugar uses it up. Chromium in most nutritional supplements is *not* highly bio-available. When you take an inorganic form of chromium such as chromium chloride, or a chromium chelated with protein, only about half of one percent ever gets into your system. Yet when it comes to energy production and management in the body, few substances are as important as chromium. When adequately supplied it helps stabilize blood sugar and ease out the mood swings that go with hypoglycaemia, keeps cholesterol low, controls appetite and reduces body fat. The most biologically active form of chromium is not elemental chromium or chromium *picolinate*, as many believe, but chromium polynicotinate in which chromium is bound to vitamin B3 (nicotinic acid) or food-state chromium (see Resources, p.137). Several studies have shown that chromium has an anabolic effect on the body. This means it helps your body build muscle so that lean body mass and muscle strength increase while body fat decreases. Athletes who use it take between 200 and 400 mcgs (micrograms) a day, depending on weight.

If when you look at your body you feel disheartened about its form, the excess of fat it carries, or the lack of tone in the flesh, forget the crash diets and take up exercise. Provided you are eating well, the right kind of exercise will not only burn off your flab, it will rebuild a good strong muscular body for you so long as you give yourself enough time to let it happen. By the way, while body building may give you magnificent muscles, only aerobic exercise can burn fat.

Slimming coffee

Coffee has a bad reputation and not without reason. A powerful stimulant to the central nervous system, caffeine taken in excess can result in increased cardiac rate, behaviourial distortions, a rise in blood fats including cholesterol, the stimulation of gastric juices leading to heartburn and interference with good digestion… the list of nasty consequences seems endless.

But, in case you think you are safe in drinking the caffeine-free version, think again. Extraction processes often rely on the action of acids, alkalis and steam or involve the use of chlorinated solvents such as *dichloromethylene*, *dichloroethylene* or *trichloroethylene*, the residues of which can be harmful to health. Even worse, the most detrimental effects of excessive coffee drinking appear to be related to the way in which coffee plantations in Third World countries are repeatedly sprayed with highly toxic pesticides – substances so dangerous they are banned in Europe and the United States. That's the bad news. At last there is good news too – especially for women wanting to shed fat.

New studies show that ordinary coffee taken before aerobic exercise actually increases the burning of body fat. It enhances your body's ability to use stored fatty acids for energy rather than glycogen stores in the muscles. Studies show, too, that caffeine significantly increases athletic performance (which is why it is now on the International Olympic Committee's list of banned substances). This is why judicious coffee drinking can be a real advantage to slimmers whose stores of glycogen are low because of calorie cutting. Caffeine actually spares your muscle tissue from being broken down for energy. This can help protect you from 'rebound' symptoms where weight in muscle is lost and then regained in fat, making you flabby. There are two keys to the correct use of coffee: take *no more than two cups* a day and only *before* doing aerobic exercise. (At any other time the caffeine is likely to disturb your insulin, bringing about rapid changes in blood-sugar levels and cravings for unhelpful foods.) Secondly, drink only freshly made organically grown coffee.

Energy magic

There is one nutritional supplement which stands out above all the rest when it comes to enhancing energy. It is a monosaccharide sugar linked to the element phosphorus called Glycophos. It provides your body's metabolic pathways with the building blocks it needs to produce the molecule ATP, which in turn is split to produce energy. Energy from the foods we eat has to go through a long and complex conversion process before it is available for use, say, to drive movement or to keep the brain functioning at peak levels. Glycophos, which comes tucked into a yeast extract and high amino-acid base, short circuits the process, enhancing energy production as well as conserving energy that the body would otherwise use up. This makes it of tremendous benefit to athletes, women in the process of shedding unwanted fat, and people who need extra brain fuel to keep going. To give you some idea of just how remarkable is Glycophos's ability to create energy, 15ml of the stuff which contains only 18 calories produces the same usable energy as almost 2 cups of peanuts with a value of 1460 calories. And it does this *cleanly* – leaving very little in the way of metabolic residues behind to clog up the works. The only catch is the stuff tastes bad. But for the athlete wanting to avoid the build up of lactic acid and anyone wanting to maintain a high-energy state that doesn't burn you out, Glycophos can be a godsend. Besides, you need very little of this remarkable liquid and its less-than-pleasant taste is masked pretty well in fruit juice (see Resources, p.136).

Fat calories are fatter

The standard patter about calories and weight gain says that all calories are the same from whatever source, and it is the quantity – not the quality – that needs to be controlled. New studies into fat metabolism show this to be completely wrong. Fat calories are a lot 'fatter' than calories from proteins or carbohydrates. The more of your calorie intake that comes from fat sources, the more likely you are to gain weight from the foods you eat no matter how much overall calorie control you exert in your diet. Masses of animal studies have demonstrated that changing to a high-fat diet (even if calorie intake remains the same as before) creates large deposits of body fat within several weeks. In a recent study one group of rats were given a diet containing forty-two per cent fat (near the average British intake of fat in humans) and another group a standard low-fat diet. Both groups were allowed to eat as much as they wanted. Over fifteen months the high-fat group actually consumed fewer calories than the low-fat group (410 as compared to 500 on average) yet they ended up with fifty-one per cent body fat. The low-fat group were far slimmer at a mere thirty per cent body fat. So far nobody is sure why this is so. It is known that fats eaten demand only one tenth of the energy to process in the body that other foods do. The energy equation, once scientists finally work it out, will probably be a great deal more complex. In the meantime if you value a flab-free body, cut down on the fats in your diet and substitute fresh vegetables and lean sources of protein.

Negative fields and positive fat loss

Another misconception which women have about exercise is that all the fat burning takes place while you are in motion. This is not the case. Some of the fat burning takes place while you exercise (particularly if you use some of the nutritional substances that encourage lipolysis like COQ and organic coffee). But, more important, exercise enhances your metabolic processes so that fat burning can occur easily while you rest as well – especially when you sleep.

Negative magnetic energy normalizes the acid/alkaline balance in the body. Used with regular aerobic exercise, sleeping in a 'magnetic bed' at night (see Chapter 11, Feeding The Core) can support your body's fat-mobilizing abilities far better than exercise alone can.

Fatty tissue is acidic. Negative magnetic fields from north pole magnets alkalinize, neutralize and *help* dissolve fatty tissues which are burnt off best in an alkaline medium. These negative fields also encourage the production of growth hormone all of which takes place at night. This is why such magnetic devices provide the latest cutting-edge technology for top athletes who want to build muscles and improve athletic performance. Unlike steroid drugs, negative magnetic fields are not only safe they are also completely legal. (No athlete has ever been banned from the Olympics for sleeping on a magnetic bed.)

Aerobic exercise during the day and sleeping on magnets at night together with conscientious food combining (see Chapter 9, Energy Grazing) is about the best lifestyle you can create for yourself to encourage your body quite naturally to readjust its fat-muscle ratios to normal.

American expert in biomagnetics, Dr William Philpott, has even had reports back from patients he has treated for various illnesses by placing strong north pole magnets (around 3500 gauss) on the abdomen, that this practice actually helps reduce fat deposits on the specific area where the magnets were placed – something which should, by rights, be impossible to do. It is, he stresses, a slow process and usually means sleeping with the magnets against the body night after night. And it won't work on its own. It is certainly no replacement for a proper lifestyle incorporating aerobic exercise and good eating. But it can be a real help to some women who, even when they shed fat and build muscle, find there are one or two areas of their bodies where resistant fat deposits remain.

The physically active lifestyle

Shed only fifty per cent of whatever excess fat you carry and you automatically increase your body energy by thirty per cent. But this takes time – time measured in terms of months and years not a mere ten days, as the latest newspaper wonder diet promises. It is, however, well worth the time and the effort it demands, for in the process not only does your whole body become rejuvenated but you also access new energy and reclaim your personal power.

But my body is ugly

One of the biggest sources of anguish for many sedentary women is the sense that they dare not *begin* to exercise because they do not want to be seen, in the shape they are in now, eased into a swimsuit or a pair of shorts. Leslie, who inherited a tendency to store fat, has never been blessed with an overabundance of self-confidence and spent many years hiding herself away and refusing to exercise. Then she learned something really important: the only way to bring about radical transformation in any situation (whether it be a relationship, emotional patterns or alterations in body shape and texture) is to *accept where you are right now.*

One of the ways of doing that is to buy yorself a pair of shorts or a swimsuit you can wear now, long before your body is the shape or texture you want it to be. Use it as a badge of self-acceptance and say to hell with the world if it thinks differently. You have every right to be as you are right *now.* You can rest assured that you will change for the better with each passing week so long as you honour your body and actually give it half a chance.

Doing this on an unconscious level gives your body *permission* to change. Without that permission (which only takes place silently in the innermost recesses of your being), you can struggle and fight and read every new article about every new technique, yet nothing fundamental and lasting in the way of transformation will happen. Bless your body with patience and kindness and acceptance. Give it the support and respect it needs, and you can watch it blossom in energy and beauty, no matter what your age and no matter what condition it may once have been in.

ONCE THE ACTIVITY BUG BITES

If exercise becomes a passion and you find yourself spending more and more of your waking hours swimming or running and training for an hour or two a day, you might consider supplementing your diet with the specific anti-oxidant nutrients your high level of activity uses up. Here are important supplements to consider:

Vitamin C	2-12gms a day
Vitamin E	200-1200Iu
Selenium	200-350mcg
Co-Enzyme Q10	30-60mg
L-glutathione	100-200mg
L-cysteine	150-300mg
L-methionine	60-120mg

Workbook
for
Energy *in*
motion

Have you ever started an exercise programme with great enthusiasm – bought a new pair of running shoes, or treated yourself to a gym subscription – only to find that several weeks later you give up? If so you're not alone. Most people who take up a new form of exercise give it up again within a few weeks. Why?

Everybody knows that exercise is supposed to be *good for you*. For many this knowledge alone provides the incentive to give it a try. So you buy the gear and dive into activity. You feel inspired and virtuous… at least for a while. Then resistance raises its ugly head. Your body aches a bit one day, the weather is bad the next, you get out of the wrong side of bed, you notice how much better the other girls in the aerobics class look in their leotards… your enthu-siasm wanes and you exercise less and less. Eventually, in spite of guilt pangs, you slip back into the 'comfort' of not exercising.

While this scenario is very common, it is also true that some women who begin to exercise stick at it. Why? Are they blessed with greater willpower? Do they not encounter resistance? Or are they just naturally more athletic? In our experience it is none of these. Anyone can develop willpower, everyone has their off days and anyone can become athletic. The real difference is that the consistent exerciser has been lucky enough to cross from the 'I should' camp of exercisers to the 'I want to' one.

Just do it

In the beginning we are all in the 'I should camp'. We have to kick-start ourselves into action and it's not easy. However, experiencing some of the benefits of exercising, such as having more energy or feeling good about yourself, can spur you on. If you continue long enough (and 'long enough' is different for everyone), one magical day you find you are actually beginning to *enjoy* yourself. Instead of dreading the next exercise session and fighting the excuses not to do it, you look forward to it. Of course this does not make you immune to resistance or excuses. And you may still stop exercising for a period of time, but because you have experienced the fun of it, something will call you back. Returning to exercise will be easier each time.

If you have exercised in the past, you may have enjoyed moments of it and know how it feels to be in the 'I want to' camp. Those of you who have never enjoyed physical activity will have to suspend your disbelief and take our word for it that *exercise can be fun*.

If you are afraid to even begin to get in shape, because you feel you are too old, too overweight or just too unfit, remember that the more impossible the challenge of becoming an exerciser seems, the more power for transformation exercise holds for you. Everyone has to begin somewhere.

Although we can't force you to take up exercise or to stick at it, we would encourage (beg, beseech!) you to try it long enough to share the experience of joy, energy and strength that it has brought us.

Make it a core choice

Unless you choose to exercise for reasons that are fundamental to your life orientation, you commit yourself only in part. The rest of you then puts up resistance in the form of excuses, which sooner or later sabotage your best intentions. On the other hand, when you make the decision to exercise from your core, you have your greatest power behind you, enabling you to override excuses and overcome any resistance you meet.

Why should I exercise?

Take a look at the following list of reasons to exercise and circle those you consider to be the 'right' ones.
1. Because it's good for me.
2. Because I enjoy it.
3. Because I'm overweight.
4. Because it lifts my spirits and helps me feel balanced emotionally.
5. Because I look awful in shorts.
6. Because it makes me feel proud of my body.
7. Because most people I know who have their act together do.
8. Because it makes me stronger – better able to cope with stress.
9. Because my friends/lover do.
10. Because it brings me a sense of confidence and self-esteem.

If you circled most of the even numbers then you have begun to understand the concept of living from the core. The odd numbered reasons are based upon external demands or expectations. They imply an 'I should,' i.e. in order to look right in a short skirt or because I have been told that it is healthy or because my friends exercise – I should. 'Should' reasons are weaker and more easily undermined because they imply in-built resistance – 'I should, but I don't really want to.' The even numbered reasons, however, all directly relate to core values such as choosing to

be whole, to be free and to trust in life. These strong reasons carry core energy and automatic willpower.

Exercise your choice

Make a list of 5 good reasons for you to exercise in your journal, then check to see if they are core reasons. Do they correspond to your deepest personal desires? Do they relate to any of the answers you made to the questions, 'Who are you?' 'What do you want?' 'What do you feel is stopping you?' in chapter 1?

Even if you have succeeded in finding only one core reason to exercise you can feel pleased. You have just taken the first step towards exercising from the core. Instead of feeling guilty about not exercising, and plaguing yourself with 'I should, but', you have cleared the way to begin.

Plan for success

Before you set foot in a training shoe, set yourself up to succeed by preparing your exercise strategy.

Pick your pleasure

Begin by choosing the right activity for you. If you love company then solitary jogging down a country lane may suit you less than joining a gym or taking a dance class with friends. If you are shy and easily discouraged by the idea of exercising in public you might be happiest working out with an exercise video in your home. There are dozens of ways to access core energy through movement. Once you become fit and confident in your body you may be inspired to try the more

adventurous or exotic activities – from rock climbing and fencing to flamenco dancing or sky diving. For the beginner who wants to make exercise a regular habit, we have found 3 forms of exercise particularly helpful because they are so simple: walking, rebounding and running.

Plan your schedule

Make an exercise schedule for the coming week. Ideally try to include at least three 30 minute sessions of your activity. Begin with 20 minutes and work up to 45 minutes or more. You may like to try a variety of activities such as an exercise class one day, walking another and swimming another. Make time for your exercise by planning in advance. Set your alarm to wake you up an hour early, for instance, or organize a childminder for an extra hour at the end of the day if needs be, so you are free to exercise.

Set your goal

Make a reasonable goal for yourself and write it down in your journal. Don't invite failure by being unrealistic. Your goal should be a challenge but not an impossibility – for instance, 'By the end of the month I want to lose 5lb' or 'In two weeks time I want to run a mile in under 9 minutes.' When you achieve your first goal, set yourself a new one.

Mark your progress

Keep an exercise log at the back of your journal in which to record your progress. Make a note of anything you notice in relation to your exercise session. In particular record any positive feedback you get such as 'My skin is clearer', 'I have more energy today' or 'I managed to walk/run all the way up the hilly bit without stopping.' Not only will this make you conscious of your progress and help you to feel proud of your achievements, but it will give you the incentive to keep going when you encounter resistance.

Chart your position

Getting fit, like getting anywhere, means knowing where you are setting out from. Use the Pulse Test (p.104) in the first part of this chapter to work out your present fitness level and establish your ideal workout range. Be sure to exercise at this level for optimal rewards. In a month's time you can retake the test to see your improvement. Another good way to see your progress is by taking a CAT scan. This technique, available at some fitness centres, measures your body fat to lean body mass ratio. It can be really inspiring for anyone who is overweight to see the that beneath their fat is a lean muscular body ready to emerge. As you become more fit, burning up excess fatty deposits, chart your success on a follow-up scan.

Paths to power
One: Walk free

Ideal for anyone who thinks she is too unfit to exercise. Although it may seem like a soft option, in fact walking is one of the very best forms of aerobic exercise. A 6-mile walk burns up only twenty per cent fewer calories than a hard run over the same distance. An excellent choice for anyone who feels low in energy or is convalescing, walking is also particularly convenient because you can incorporate it into your daily routine to get you from A to B.

To begin with decide to walk for 30 minutes a day at a pace where your breathing becomes heavy but not strained. Make sure you wear comfortable clothes and good walking shoes. If you walk to work you can carry another pair of shoes with you to change into. After a week of walking for 30 minutes a day, go a step further. Try walking for an hour and see how far you get. As a guideline you should be able to manage 3 miles in an hour at a leisurely pace or 3 1/2 at a brisker one. As you become stronger you might like to try hill-walking or even running.

Two: Bounce into shape

Rebounding is the perfect solution for anyone who wants to exercise at home, no matter what her fitness level. Unlike many in-the-home exercise options, rebounding has a particularly high continued use success rate. In case you are unfamiliar with the term, it means bouncing up and down on a mini-trampoline. We love it as an alternative to running during bad weather. Apart from being fun in the most natural childlike way, rebounding has some extraordinary health benefits thanks to the forces of gravity exerted on you as you bounce. At the top of each bounce for a split-second gravity is non-existent. You experience weightlessness like an astronaut in space. At the bottom of a bounce, gravity is increased by 2 to 3 times its normal force. This rhythmic pressure on each of your body's cells stimulates the lymphatic system to eliminate stored wastes – the type of wastes which incidentally are responsible for cellulite. Rebounding is not only great for newcomers to exercise but is also often used by athletes as part of their training programme – particularly to repair and rebuild muscles after an injury.

Begin bouncing gently so that your heels barely leave the ground. If you feel unsteady, use the back of a chair to support yourself with one arm as you bounce. You might like to bounce to music or even while watching your favourite television programme. As an alternative to bouncing with both feet together, try jogging from one foot to the other. Begin with 10 to 15 minutes a day and work up to 30 minutes or so as your strength increases. You can also do various exercises on the rebounder to work the muscles throughout your body (see Resources, p.137, for suppliers).

Three: Run to freedom

Ideal for anyone who is keen to experience the high-energy benefits of regular exercise quickly. Although running along a beach or in a forest is a totally different experience from pounding concrete city pavements, we have enjoyed both over long periods of time. Running is perhaps the most adaptable and practical of all forms of exercise. For anyone who travels often it can be ideal. Running shoes, shorts, a teeshirt and running bra (plus a thin waterproof top and Walkman if you like) take up minimal space in a suitcase. You can also run almost anytime and anywhere.

Since it first became popular, running or jogging has received some bad press with claims that it provokes back problems and other injuries. We feel that any small problems are far outweighed by the good it does for us. We minimize injuries by wearing a decent pair of running shoes (not any old plimsolls) and stretching out for 5-10 minutes after running. Some of the simple yoga postures are ideal as a 'warm down' for keeping your muscles supple.

Begin by making a circuit for yourself of about a mile. Start out slowly and jog as far as you can. Don't push yourself so hard that you are breathless. At the right pace you should still be able to carry on a conversation as you jog. If you do find you get out of breath, alternate running with walking. Above all be patient. After a week or two, see if you can run the whole mile. When this becomes easy, increase your distance until you can run 2 or 3 miles. If you are really ambitious you might like to try a marathon. Experts claim that once you can run for 45 minutes you can begin to train for one.

Grab some incentive

- Find a picture of your chosen activity or an inspiring quotation (we like 'Just Do It') and pin it up on your bathroom mirror and fridge for encouragement.
- Before you go to bed at night, give yourself a pep talk about your activity the following day and envisage yourself enjoying it.
- Lay your exercise clothes out ready for the next day. Many runners agree that the hardest part of a morning run is putting their shoes on and stepping out of the door. After that it's easy.
- Make a deal with a good friend to get fit together. Sharing the challenge of reclaiming body power with a friend is much more fun. (It can also give you a chance to moan and sympathize over aches and pains.)
- If you choose walking or running as your activity, borrow or buy a dog to accompany you. Dogs have endless enthusiasm for walks and runs (however bad the weather).
- Hunt for a good coach or teacher – especially if you choose to work out at a gym or take an exercise class. The right one can provide encouragement and motivation.

You are bound to encounter resistance at some point in the form of injuries, bad weather, illness, or disruption of your routine due to other commitments. Don't chastise yourself and feel guilty about not exercising or breaking your programme. Simply set yourself a date to begin afresh. Read back over the positive feedback in your exercise log, draw upon the incentives above and ease back into activity.

Personal experience

Every woman who gets hooked on exercise has a unique experience of it. Some like Leslie take up exercise in very bad shape after 10 years or more of inactivity. Others, like Susannah, get back into physical activity after forgetting for only a short while how great it makes you feel. Here is what our own experience has been:

Leslie: painful progress

My favourite aerobic sport is running. One of the main reasons I was determined to try it was that running was the one sports activity I was no good at at school. Running my first mile was the hardest thing I have ever done in my life. That was 15 years ago. So you can see I have quite literally developed a passion for it.

I decided to run because I had read all about the psychological benefits of running and because, after several years of being something of a lounge lizard, I felt I needed to get fit somehow. I began one cold November morning at 5 a.m. It was the only time, apart from the middle of the night, when I could be relatively sure that there would be practically nobody on the roads. I did *not* want to be seen. Mustering all the courage I could, I made a dash through the front door, up the drive, and along the street. I went about 50 yards before I felt that I would die from the exertion and had to stop and walk.

It wasn't my legs, it was my lungs – I just couldn't get enough air. I walked panting for another 50 yards or so and then resumed my jog. I found I could just sustain the running for about the distance between one set of lamp posts, then I would walk between the next set. In this way I finally completed my circuit – the mile distance (I had measured it by driving it in my car) around a large cemetery near my house and then home again. I arrived home exhausted, dispirited and depressed.

The next day I found a hundred reasons why (no matter what all those books said about running) I should *not* repeat my performance. But something, I'm not sure what, had got hold of me. And when 5a.m. came around again there I was, with aching hips and ankles, ready to submit myself to the same torture. I did just as badly.

Three or 4 days later, to my amazement, I found I could run between *two* sets of lamp posts before having to walk the next set. Ten days later, somehow – with tears streaming down my cheeks and curses at my own stupidity for taking up such an absurd activity – I actually ran a mile. I couldn't believe that it had happened. I had the same desire to stop and walk several times but for some reason I didn't. I kept saying to myself, 'Just a little farther and then I'll stop' – but when a 'little farther' came I pushed on again and again.

When I finally arrived home, instead of being pleased with my triumph, I had the feeling that I hadn't really done it, that I had made it all up the way a child tells a story about what she has done at school today. Or that my having run a mile was an accident of fate I would never be able to repeat.

But fate was with me, and I did repeat it the next day and the day after. Soon I was running 2 miles a day and then, one wintry morning about 6 weeks after my first painful attempt, to my amazement I found I actually *enjoyed* it. I don't mean just the feeling afterwards when you have pushed yourself hard, your face is flushed, and you feel alive and good. I mean the actual running. There was something about it that was wonderful to me. In a fit of exuberance I scribbled down my experience:

This morning I ran along a road
where I had run before:
Yet I saw things which I had
  never seen.
Legs heavy, breathing hard, my
heart was light.
My body was full of life.
Then it began to rain.
Such joy.

I had caught the running bug, which everyone I have ever read on running warns will happen sooner or later, and I wasn't going to give it up. Oh, there have been days here and there when I lie in bed and convince myself that running is a bore and that I am too tired, too busy or too something else to go out that day. Some days I've indulged my laziness but never for long because, to my amazement, my love of the bed (which has always been very great indeed) doesn't seem to come up to my love of being on the road. So the next day I put on my running shoes and I'm off again.

I've found out a lot about myself and a lot about living from my hours on the road. I've learned that I am capable of succeeding at things I never thought I could accomplish. I have gained a better sense of my own strengths and my own limitations. I have grown thinner, firmer, fitter and happier. I've rediscovered the fun of play, the idea of doing something for its own sake – an art that I had long ago forgotten. Running has also given me more physical and mental perseverance. Where before I was always inclined to give up when things got difficult, now, although I'm just as *inclined* to give up, I do it far less often because I have found out that if you concentrate on putting one foot in front of the other you can get there – wherever 'there' happens to be at that moment. Most important, I have learned that you have to go through discipline to obtain freedom.

It may be the commonsense of the common man to consent to be ordinary, but now, everything instinctive, everything intuitive, everything beyond logic tells me otherwise. It tells me that compared to what I *ought* to be, I am only half

awake. It tells me, as William James did, that I am using only a small part of my mental and physical resources. Running gave me these insights. It made me an athlete, albeit an ageing one, and started my ascent towards a new goal…

Susannah: back on track

Although as a teenager I was quite athletic and enjoyed running throughout university, I found that living in a city began to dampen my enthusiasm for exercise. Having to put up with traffic fumes, red lights, bad weather and knee injuries eventually put a stop to my running. Before I realized it I had gone for a couple of years with almost no exercise, apart from a few dance classes or the occasional family softball game. At a particularly stressful time in my life I decided I needed the support exercise had afforded me.

At the time I shared a flat with a girl called Karen who swam at an indoor pool every day. I knew swimming was one of the best forms of all-round exercise, and so I decided to give it a try. I thought it might be fun. It wasn't. I hated it. I felt flabby in my swimsuit. The chlorine stank. There were too many people and having to swim laps bored me. I left the pool with messy hair and bloodshot eyes, feeling exhausted and discouraged, 'Forget swimming,' I thought, 'I'll try something else.'

I noticed that Karen felt differently about it. I saw how she organized her day around swimming so that, even if it was last thing at night, after work, or during her lunch hour, she would still manage to get to the pool. I couldn't believe that anyone could be so disciplined. When I told her that I envied her iron discipline she laughed, 'It's not discipline at all,' she told me, 'I just love to swim.'

Determined to see how that was possible in a gloomy city pool (and inspired by Karen's contagious enthusiasm), I decided I would give it a try for one week. I bought myself a decent pair of goggles and a swimming cap, found a comfortable cotton swimsuit, and made a "kit bag" with sample-sized bottles of shampoo, conditioner and moisturizer, plus some make-up, which I could carry around with me, so that I could swim whenever I got the chance during the day and leave the pool looking acceptable. Each day I gritted my teeth and forced myself to the pool to swim my laps. I tried to make the routine as brief and bother-free as possible. At the end of the week I noticed that rather than being a burden, my routine was beginning to be fun. Instead of being bored by swimming lengths I became excited by the challenge of how well and how fast I could do them. I had always wanted to learn to do butterfly – it reminds me of the way a dolphin swims. My secret attempts (in deserted pools) more closely resembled the floundering of a walrus. After a while I plucked up courage and enrolled in a swimming improvement class. After a couple of weeks, to my amazement, I began to get the knack of it. Pretty soon I could not only swim a few strokes but even breathe! Then I could swim half a length, then a length. The feeling of weaving through the water was so wonderful that I couldn't wait to get back in the water each day. Exercise had finally become something I *wanted* to do.

The pool has become a second home. I have made friends there who inspire me on the days when I lack incentive. One man – an air steward – swims for 3 hours at a time. Whenever I feel tired or wonder whether I can manage my 30-45 minutes (or worry that I might be overdoing it) I think of him and just get on with it. When I am travelling and can't get to a pool (or a lake or the sea), I run instead. I am sure there will be periods where I forget the joys of exercise and go off track again, but I hope always to find my way back.

Turn flab to force

Women tend to build up excess fat in 3 common areas: the buttocks, stomach and thighs. Even with regular aerobic exercise, the fat in these areas can be hard to shed. Too many women go around hating their flabby thighs or sagging bottom. Some even subject themselves to gruelling 'killer aerobics' in an attempt to pummel the offending body parts into shape. This common attitude of disgust for fat only separates a woman further from her body.

Look upon your excess fat, cellulite or sagging muscles as an indication that a particular part of your body has lost its power and needs help to regain it. Feed weak areas with strengthening exercises to reclaim your body's full power.

Power toning

In addition to aerobic exercise, we use the following exercise routine, based on the Pilates technique taught to us by expert Alan Herdman, to keep the stomach, buttocks and thighs trim. In just 10-15 minutes a day these simple exercises, together with the advice in the previous chapter, can help sculpt away excess fat, leaving your body strong and toned.

Breathe in awareness

The Power Toning exercises are twice as effective when you do them with awareness. By consciously directing your attention and breath to an area of your body as you work it, you can bring the power of your mind into play. As you will remember from Chapter 3, Free Your Spirit, conscious thought has an impressive and often unrecognized influence on physical matter. The combination of physically exerting your muscles, together with mentally inviting awareness to them is powerfully transformative.

NB: Remember to breathe out during the most strenuous part of the exercise, and in on the recovery. If you are doing a leg lift, for instance, breathe out as you lift the leg against gravity and in as you lower it again. Don't push yourself too hard. Instead work with kindness. Try for 10 repetitions of each in the beginning. As your muscles get stronger, you can increase the repetitions to 20 or more.

Stomach I

Lie on your back with your arms by your sides. Lift your knees into your chest and then stretch your legs up towards the ceiling, toes pointed. Now lift your shoulders and chest off the floor, stretching your hands away from you along the floor. Keeping your chin tucked into your chest, squeeze your buttocks and inner thighs together. Now begin beating the floor with your hands. Breathe in for 4 beats and out for 4 – count 1. Then breathe in again for 4 and out for 4 and count 2 and so forth up to 10. Then rest, hugging your knees to your chest.

More advanced: hold your legs at 60° to the floor instead of 90°, turn your thighs out, flex your feet and squeeze the thighs together.

Stomach II

Lie on your back as in Stomach I. Lift your legs to the ceiling, toes pointed. Lift your chest off the floor, this time reaching your arms at an angle of about 60° to the floor (or think of reaching your hands to the corner where the wall in front of you meets the ceiling.) Holding this position with your upper body, lower one leg towards the floor until it almost touching, then bring it back up. Repeat with the other leg. Do 5-10 with each leg and rest.

More advanced: as with Stomach I, hold your highest leg at 60° instead of 90°.

Waist refiner stretch

Stand or sit with legs astride. With your hands clasped behind your head stretch over to one side for a count of 10, then to the other side. Repeat 2-3 times on each side.

Waist lifts

Lie on your side with your head resting on your elbow and your other hand in front of your chest on the floor for balance. Keeping your body in a straight line, legs stretched out and toes pointed, lift both feet off the ground as high as poss-

ible and lower again. Repeat 10-20 times on each side. NB: Don't be discouraged, this exercise is hard!

Leg lifts I

Lie on your side in a straight line as for Waist Lifts. (If you have trouble balancing, lie with your back against a wall.) Rest yourself on the forearm of your underneath arm, with your hand pointing either in front of you or towards your head. Place your other hand on your upper hip. Bend your underneath leg to a comfortable angle. Stretch your upper leg with the foot flexed and lift it up to about 8 inches above your hip, then lower. Make sure you lift only the leg, not the hip, by using your upper hand to keep your hip still. Repeat 10-20 times on each leg.

Leg lifts II

Lie on your side as for Leg Lifts I. This time bend your upper leg and place your foot comfortably in front of your knee or thigh. Place your underneath forearm along the floor as in Leg Lift I, but place your other hand in front of you on the floor for support. Now lift the underneath leg up, toe pointed, and lower. Repeat 10-20 times on each leg.

Leg lifts III

Lie on your side, supported on your forearm as in Leg Lifts I. Place your upper hand on the floor in front of your chest for balance. Bend your underneath knee to a comfortable angle. Now stretch your upper leg, lifting it to the side, about hip level, then swing it forward in front of you to an angle of 90° to your body. Now lift the leg up about 6 inches and lower again to hip level in front

of you. Lift and lower in this position 10-20 times and then return the leg to the side and lower. Repeat with other leg.

Leg lifts IV

Lie on your stomach, supporting your upper body on your forearms, looking ahead of you. With your feet about 8 inches apart, straighten your legs, turn your thighs out and squeeze your buttocks together. Now lift one leg at a time, pulling your stomach muscles up towards your head to support your lower back. Repeat 10 times on each leg.

Thigh lifts

Kneeling up on your hands and knees, stomach lifted, swing one leg out to the side, keeping the knee bent, so that the lifted knee forms a right angle with the one supporting you, and then lower. Repeat 10-20 times with each leg.

For a more difficult variation, after lifting the knee to the side, keep it lifted and move it around to the back as far as possible, then return it to the side position. Move it back and to the side each time. Repeat 10-20 times on each leg.

Cushion squeeze

Lie on your back with your knees bent, feet together, soles flat to the floor. Place a cushion between your knees. Press your lower back to the floor and squeeze your knees together for a count of 5 seconds. Then relax. Repeat 5-10 times. Finally, with the cushion squeezed between your knees, contract and release your buttock muscles, lifting your pelvis just slightly off the floor as you do. Repeat 10-20 times.

Chapter 11

Feeding *the* core

Being able to call on endless energy depends on how well you feed your core – physically, emotionally and spiritually – day by day. This means developing a lifestyle which incorporates exercise, good food, restorative sleep and the myriad of other possible factors, from magnetic beds to meditation, that help support your own brand of vitality at peak efficiency. When creating such a lifestyle for yourself there is one simple but essential thing to remember: your body *is* energy. What your body most certainly is *not* is some dense physical object you have to bolster up or beat into submission so it can keep going.

The body as energy

Practically everything that is written about the body in terms of exercise, nutrition and health-supporting treatments gets hung up on the outdated mechanical worldview which ignores this. The standard advice leaves out the fact that every physical and chemical change that takes place in your body is really a *secondary* effect of some *primary* energy change. Learning a little about what influences your body as a unified energetic system and beginning to think in this way enables you to call on simple yet potent energy-enhancing, energy-altering and energy-supporting practices that can make everything in your life a lot easier.

Take one rat dead or alive

More than sixty years ago, a brilliant scientist, Albert Szent-Gyorgyi, used to ask a simple question at dinner parties: 'What is the difference between a living rat and a dead one?' According to the laws of classical chemistry and physics, based on the old worldview, there is no fundamental difference. Yet as any fool can see this is rubbish. Szent-Gyorgyi's own reply was simple yet revolutionary – 'Some kind of electricity.'

Winner of two Nobel prizes for his work, he had years before observed that the molecular structure of a living cell somehow acts as a semiconductor for electromagnetic or magnetic energy. Semiconduction takes place only in materials which have a highly ordered structure, such as crystals, in which the atoms are arranged in neat geometrical lattices. This enables electrons to move with ease from the orbit of one molecule to another. It is the ease with which electron transfer occurs that largely determines the experience of *aliveness* both in an individual cell and in the body as a whole.

Other eminent scientists before Szent-Gyorgyi such as American surgeon George Crile, engineer Georges Lakhovsky and physician Harold Saxton Burr also explored the nature of living things from an energetic point of view. But it was not until an outstanding American orthopaedic surgeon Robert O. Becker came along that a real understanding of the energy control system in the human body began to be understood.

Energy control starts here

Becker postulated that an analogue-coded electronic information system exists in the body which carries energetic information to regulate cell division and healing, and to support life processes. This system, he theorized, may even be the interface by which thoughts are able to induce physical and biochemical changes in the human body (how spiritual healing works, for instance, and creative visualization used for healing and for improving sports performance).

Putting his theory into practice with animal studies, Becker discovered that such a system does indeed exist. It has regulating, self-organizing and self-repairing properties based on semiconductivity and it is strongly influenced for good or ill by magnetic and electromagnetic fields. So Becker began to use minute electrical currents to produce electromagnetic fields that speed the healing of tissues and bones, with excellent results. For this work he was twice nominated for a Nobel prize. He then went on to explore the way in which the 'information' from magnetic and electromagnetic fields affects human beings for good or ill and to caution that many electromagnetic influences in day to day life (see p.44) can be highly detrimental to health.

This may all sound highfalutin and super-scientific, but it is important. Because once you get the sense of your body as energy and learn how to support that energy with such things as exercise, loving care, and even perhaps the use of solid state magnets, this can help you break through forever the sense of separation from your body which makes a woman prey to feelings of inadequacy and powerlessness.

The body magnetic

Every cell in your body has a positive (north-seeking) and a negative (south-seeking) pole. So do direct electrical currents, magnets and even the earth itself. In fact every living organism is largely made up of charged particles such as electrons, protons, and ions like calcium, sodium and potassium, or paramagnetic particles such as neutrons, all of which look after the biological functions that keep you alive. It is also true of groups of cells. Your central nervous system is electromagnetic positive in its polarity while peripheral areas of your body are electromagnetic negative. It is this difference in potential or charge that makes the energy flow in the body. *This*, and this alone, is the difference between Szent-Gyorgyi's live rat and his dead one.

Human physical and mental energy are both in essence *magnetic* energy which your body produces and accesses in many different ways. Much of it comes from the foods you eat and the water you drink. Other things can transfer energy to us, too, like light entering through the eye, or sound, or ionizers, or essential oils, or colour, or thought. All of these in one form or another transmit electromagnetic *information* to which our body's own magnetic fields respond. When there is enough light in your environment, and it is full spectrum, like the light you get from the sun, it feeds core energy and helps you look and feel great. When there is too little light, or when you spend long hours working under tungsten bulbs or flickering fluorescent tubes indoors, it can give you the blues or even result in what is now called SAD (Seasonal Affective Disorder).

Earth pulse

Magnetic energy is one of the most powerful forces in the universe. The earth has a natural pulsed frequency of 7.96 cycles per second. Investigations into the effects of magnetic fields on the human body, in an attempt to keep astronauts in good condition, have shown that when humans are subjected to this natural pulsed frequency (provided it is of sufficient gauss strength) their stress levels fall, they sleep well and maintain a fine emotional balance. For optimal health – mental, emotional and spiritual – the body needs a good supply of negative magnetic energy at the proper frequency.

This usable supply of energy supports the core superbly. The trouble is, because of the ubiquitous electromagnetic pollution present on the earth as a result of manmade electromagnetic fields from power lines, radar, microwaves, satellites, ham radios and even electrical appliances, we are all forced to live in an environment in which the electromagnetic *information* reaching the body has become highly distorted. This high-frequency energy causes our cells to go out of resonance, fatiguing them, which drains the body's natural core energy instead of supporting it.

Another factor comes into things too – the *strength* of fields. Magnetic fields are measured in units of energy called *gauss*. Research in geophysics has shown that the gauss strength of the earth's natural magnetic field has decreased dramatically. Four thousand years ago it was approximately 4 gauss. Today, on average, it is a mere 0.4 gauss, varying somewhat from one location to another. Studying the effects of this decrease in the late 1950s, Japanese scientists reported for the first time that a new syndrome was appearing in human beings. They dubbed it *magnetic field deficiency syndrome*. It is characterized by lack of energy, insomnia, general aches and pains, stiffness, frequent headaches, constipation and so forth. Yet most people are unaware that these symptoms can be environmentally caused by a deficient geomagnetic field.

Dissipating energy

Positive and negative magnetic influences produce quite distinct effects on the body. When exposure to positive magnetic energy is greater than negative it tends to overstimulate human metabolism. When negative magnetic energy exceeds positive it normalizes metabolism. Your life energy is burnt up each day in activity. It is also drained by internal stressors and depleted by exposure to external aggressors in the environment. All of this can throw things out of balance. So you suffer.

The common usage of the word 'negative' brings to mind something undesirable or unfavourable. This is not the case when it comes to 'negative' electricity and magnetism. The negative pole has a surplus of negatively charged electrons – good available energy. The positive pole is defined as a deficiency of electrons. An increase in electrons means an increase in energy.

Unfortunately modern urban life, with all its emotional pressures and external aggressors tips the balance sharply towards the positive magnetic energy side with its fatiguing too-high frequency.

The good news is that there is a lot you can do to

POSITIVE AND NEGATIVE MAGNETICS

Negative fields	Positive fields
Increase oxygen in the cells	Decrease oxygen in cells
Encourage restful sleep	Stimulate the body
Counter infection	Encourage bacterial growth
Encourage fat-burning	Encourage the build up of fat
Enhance mental functions	Cause mental overactivity
Relieve stress symptoms	Intensify stress symptoms
Encourage contentment	Encourage depression
Encourage repair and healing	Slow down repair and healing
Relieve pain	Increase pain

counter the negative effects of excessive exposure to positive magnetic fields. Using full-spectrum lighting, harmonious sound from instruments such as wind chimes, meditation, colour to create an environment for yourself at work and home, a diet of natural foods, as well as magnetic health-supporting devices, all help feed core energy instead of draining or distorting it. Also many chronic conditions, both mental and physical, can be alleviated by the application of solid state unipoled magnets of the right sort and strength directly onto the body.

Solid state health

American psychiatrist William Philpott MD is considered an expert in the English-speaking world on positive and negative magnetic fields applied to the human body. He has successfully treated more than 7000 patients in the USA for illnesses as diverse as depression, anxiety neurosis and psychosis, arthritis, allergies, diabetes and chronic fatigue using solid state magnets.

He has found that negative magnetic fields transferred to the body from magnets encourage regenerative sleep, banish pain, help to heal cuts and broken bones, dissolve calcium deposits around arthritic joints, fight infection and increase oxygenation in the cells, creating greater vitality in the body as a whole. They help strengthen the immune system against illness and premature ageing. Used regularly, they can also help people maintain a balanced emotional life.

Another expert in biomagnetics, Dean Bonlie, has helped many top athletes in the USA and Canada to improve their performance by getting them to sleep on mattresses containing magnets which subject the body to a steady negative magnetic field night after night. He believes that by placing the body's charged and paramagnetic particles in a steady-state negative magnetic field, there is an increase in the orbital energy of these particles. This is reflected in faster, more efficient biochemical reactions and more rapid diffusions of gases and ions through cellular membranes, both of which would appear to enhance human performance. This is demonstrated by up to twenty per cent increases in performance and eighty per cent reduction in soreness after major workouts by athletes using these beds.

Beware of cowboys

This science of biomagnetics is already revolutionizing diagnostic instruments in medicine. It has led to the development of nuclear magnetic resonance imaging (MRI) which is more effective than x-rays in soft-tissue diagnosis without the risk of radiation, magnetoencephalograms (MEG) for diagnosing brain disorders, magnetocardiograms (MKG) to assist in heart condition diagnosis, and superconducting quantum interference conductors (SQUID) which identify and measure minute magnetic fields in living organisms. Within the next quarter of a century, the use of health-enhancing negative magnetic fields from solid state magnets placed on the body and the practice of sleeping on magnetic beds is, we believe, going to revolutionize self-care too. But let the buyer beware. There are many cowboys more knowledgeable about sales techniques than they are about magnetic fields, trying to get in on the act. They sell products, from magnetic beds and futons to devices for knee pain and tennis elbow, which don't work. Either their gauss strength is too low, the magnets are the wrong kind or they create positive magnetic fields which do not benefit the body long term. Even many Japanese products, which you would expect to be good, create both positive and negative fields. Mixed magnetic fields may help temporarily but they only exacerbate things in the long run. If you decide to make magnets or a magnetic bed part of your own lifestyle, buy only those which have been scientifically designed and properly made (see Resources, p.137).

Core energy at its best

To create the best possible environment for supporting core energy, fill your life, your home and, as much as possible, your work environment with everything that is life-giving. Sound, colour, light and charged ions in the atmosphere all make measurable shifts in your magnetic energy. These and other things can soothe and restore a system that has been physically and emotionally jangled by a harsh environment. They help counteract the chemical and emotional pollution which are subjected to.

MAGIC MATTRESSES AND OTHER MAGNETICS

Here are some useful ways to use solid state unipoled magnets.

Blissful sleep
Use a 'magnetic' bed – a mattress filled with unipole magnets with a surface gauss strength above 1000, made with around 3" of cushioning material for comfort and to distance your body from the positive field between the magnets. The mattress should be the same size as your bed frame and the negative side of the magnetic mattress (north-pole means south-seeking) should always face the body. This not only gets rid of aches and pains and helps overcome sleeplessness, it also helps create emotional balance, mental clarity and increases vitality. It even encourages the secretion of growth hormone which helps keep the body young, can improve the look and shape of the body, and can enhance athletic performance.

Help for sore heads
Put a unipole 4" x 6" ceramic magnet (surface gauss strength 1100) or a couple of smaller ceramic cube magnets (surface gauss strength 1100) over the painful area with the negative side towards the skin. If there is no change within a few minutes, you can try the magnet on the opposite side of the head.

Protection from VDUs
Wear a 3" x 3" plastic magnet (gauss 200-2500) over your heart area when using a VDU to help protect yourself from electromagnetic radiation. (We wear such a magnet on aeroplanes too and when we are in cities to help us keep our cool in the midst of frantic environments.) Philpott explains that, because all the blood flows through the heart area, and negative magnetic fields help cleanse the body of wastes and oxygenate the cells, this practice can be helpful to balance, energy and wellbeing.

Sports injuries
Rest the injured area on the negative side of a unipoled 4" x 6" x 1" ceramic magnet for as much time as possible during the early stages after an injury. The magnet may be wrapped in a soft cloth for more comfort if necessary. For more mobility, place a 1" x 2" x ¾" unipoled block ceramic magnet with the negative side to the injury and hold it in place with tape or a crepe bandage. Wear it at night to reduce swelling and inflammation.

Workbook *for* Feeding *the* core

In Chapter 5, Weeding Out the Blockers and Drainers, we looked at all the things, both outer and inner, which inhibit or deplete your energy. Now let's look at the energy enhancers and see what resources are available for feeding core energy. These enhancers can be internal – techniques like meditation or guided imagery which help to restore and balance the body. Or they can be external – such as the practices which allow you to draw upon the life energy in concentrated plant essences or sunlight. Both the inner and outer energy-enhancers are important to provide your core with the most supportive environment possible.

External enhancers

As the world gets more polluted, the prospect of creating the life-nurturing 'cocoon' of our home environment becomes increasingly appealing. There are many ways to do this. You can draw upon the power of nature to revitalize you, in the form of hydrotherapy and aromatherapy practices, or charge your environment with energy that mimics the benefits of nature at her best – ionizers, full-spectrum lights, therapeutic magnets and energy-balancing sounds, fragrances, fabrics and colours.

Colour affects you
Colour it beautiful

The therapeutic use of colour dates as far back as the first century AD when the famous Roman physician Celsus prescribed medicines of specific colours to treat different ailments. Recent research by Dr Alexander Schauss, Director of the American Institute for Biosocial Research, has confirmed the physiological effects of colour on the mind and body. Light energy from a coloured object is absorbed by the photoreceptors in the retina of the eye and converted into electrical energy. This travels to the brain via nerve impulses and stimulates the pituitary and pineal glands. Together these glands regulate several of the body's physiological systems. Because each colour sends a slightly different electrical message to the brain, each affects us in a different way.

Mind/body colours
- **Red** Stimulating – excites and warms the body, increases heart rate, brain activity and respiration.
- **Pink** Soothing – relaxes the muscles, subdues aggression and anxiety, encourages rest.
- **Orange** Stimulating – encourages appetite and reduces fatigue.
- **Yellow** Energizing – stimulates the memory, increases pulse rate and lifts the spirits.
- **Green** Uplifting – relieves depression, soothes and relaxes both mind and body.
- **Blue** Relaxing – lowers blood pressure, heart rate and respiration; soothes and 'cools' the emotions.

Looking at colour this way can help you create the most appropriate and beneficial colour environments in your home. When decorating your living space, consider which colour qualities are best for a particular room. Short of painting it, a great way to add colour to a room is to make a simple frame of plywood and stretch a piece of coloured fabric across it, then use it as a wall hanging. You can also play with colour in the way you dress. If you need energy, for instance, go for the warmer colours – red, orange and yellow. Colour is only one part of cocoon making; equally important are all the things you can do to bring the atmosphere of, say, a beautiful country meadow to a small city flat.

From city to country

Being out in nature – walking in the mountains or relaxing on a warm beach – helps restore you mentally and physically. Anyone who has to spend most of her time in a city environment deprived of health-supporting natural elements can create them for herself.

Make some green friends

House plants can make your home or office environment more friendly and even more healthy. Apart from their uplifting appearance, green plants are also natural air purifiers. Thanks to photosynthesis, they supply a room with fresh oxygen during the daylight hours. Even more important, they can remove toxic organic pollutants from the air. A study by NASA and the Associated Landscape Contractors of America showed that 14 common house plants have air-purifying properties. The common Ficus, for instance, removes fifty per cent of the formaldehyde in air. Formaldehyde is a common household pollutant found in chemicals used in the manufacture of carpets and permanent press sheets as well as composition wood furniture. The study showed that the leaves of the plants were responsible for up to 20% of the plant's purifying properties while the roots and soil microbes accounted for the rest. As a guide, one 12" potted plant can clean the air of a 10' x 10' room.

Sleep with a sea breeze

Breathing the air on a mountainside or near the sea makes you feel uplifted and well – 'Ah, good fresh air!' we say. What we are reacting to is the abundance of negatively charged air molecules in each breath. In the city, air pollutants, concrete structures, synthetic fabrics and plastic interiors all conspire to deplete these negatively charged molecules. This results in a predominance of positively charged ions or even a depletion of all ions. As a result we can suffer from fatigue, depression and hypertension as well as migraine headaches, allergies and respiratory disorders. A wonderful manmade antidote to polluted air comes in the form of an ionizer – a device which negatively charges air particles. Using one at your office or beside your bed at night can soothe away stress and help you to breathe easy (see Resources, p.137).

Enjoy an air bath

The air bath is the easiest of the 'nature cure' treatments. It involves simply removing your clothes and allowing fresh air to circulate around your body for a few minutes at a time. Giving your skin a chance to breathe in this way, unrestricted by clothing, can enhance the body's metabolism and balance body energies. The simplest way to enjoy an air bath is to strip down while you do your morning or evening toilette. Open a window in the bathroom so that there is fresh air. Turn on a heater if the room is too chilly, although cool air for a few minutes can have a stimulating and strengthening effect on the system.

Let the sunshine in

The sun's rays, much maligned for their role in the premature ageing of the skin and skin cancer, are also responsible for all life energy on our planet. Without sunlight we would not exist. With insufficient exposure to the sun we suffer. Sunlight plays an important role in several vital physiological functions. UV rays from the sun act directly on the skin, stimulating the production of vitamins A and D. This in turn facilitates the absorption of calcium into the bones. These same rays also stimulate the production of sex hormones, help lower high blood pressure and strengthen the immune system. Sunlight shining through the eyes also regulates our biological clock, sleep patterns and moods by stimulating the body's hormonal and neurochemical controls via the hypothalamus and pineal glands. In short, along with water, food and oxygen, sunlight is essential to healthy human life. So wear a good sunscreen, leave the dark glasses off and get out in it often.

The safe sun bath

The best way to get your daily dose of sunlight is to sunbathe outdoors for carefully controlled periods of time – exposing as much naked skin as possible. This can be done even in winter if you can find an area that is sufficiently sheltered from the wind. And even if the day seems grey and overcast, you can still benefit from the sun's influence. In the summer you should sunbathe only before 11a.m. or after 3p.m. when the sun is not at its strongest. Start with as little as 2 minutes on each part of your body – front, back, left side and right side in full summer sun, then gradually lengthen your time by a minute on each area working up to 10 or 15 minutes on each part per day. This kind of gentle sun exposure, unlike grilling your skin for hours at a time on a sunny beach, will allow you to capitalize on the benefits and avoid the harm of excessive exposure. We strongly recommend the use of a total sunscreen on your face whenever you are exposed to sunlight. A moisturizer with UVA and UVB filters is adequate during the low-sun winter months. Otherwise you need a screen with a protection factor of at least 8. The rest of your body should also be protected from strong sunlight with a good suntan oil or lotion appropriate to your skin type.

Another way to get your daily dose of beneficial sun is during an outdoors exercise session. Aerobic exercise complements the sun's beneficial effects, heightening mood and improving stamina and muscle tone. Little wonder that the ancient Romans trained their finest gladiators in full sunlight.

Sunlight in a box

If you spend a good deal of time working in an artificially lit indoor environment you may be deprived of adequate sunlight. Artificial light in the home and workplace not only lacks the important UVA

and UVB rays but also amounts to only one-tenth of the strength of natural light (even on a dull day) – 500 lux indoors compared to 5,000 lux outdoors. Anyone who suffers the symptoms of sunlight deficiency, which can include severe depression, fatigue, and increased appetite and weight gain, can benefit from bringing the sunlight indoors by installing full-spectrum lighting where they live and work or by using a full-spectrum 'light box' every day. Artificial full-spectrum lights simulate about 90% of the components of natural sunlight, including the UV frequencies. Just a few hours of exposure to them each day has been shown to relieve symptoms of light deficiency in 80% of the cases tested, within only 5 days (see Resources p.136).

Heaven scent

Both your ability to smell and your experience of intense emotions such as joy, fear, desire or rage are governed by the most primitive part of your brain – the limbic system. That is probably why a particular smell – an ex-lover's aftershave, grandma's apple pie – can be so emotionally evocative. Each time you detect a particular smell you are reacting to volatile molecules of odour wafting their way to odour receptors at the ends of millions of nerve cells located behind the bridge of your nose. From there nerve impulses are carried to the limbic system where the messages are interpreted and where responses are mediated via the hypothalamus to the rest of your body.

Not only does scent affect you emotionally but also physiologi-

cally thanks to the 'messages' which specific odour molecules carry to your brain. Some of the most powerful message carriers come in the form of aromatic plant oils – the distilled essences of various plants' leaves, fruits, flowers, bark and roots, which are literally brimming over with the structural information of life. Many people are aware of the use of essential oils in pleasant aromatherapy massage, but few realize that similar high-quality plant essences, expertly selected and extracted, are also administered both internally and externally by medical doctors in the treatment of serious physical and mental disorders.

Each aromatic essence carries a different message to the body: vanilla and lavender, for instance, tell the body to relax, while peppermint and rosemary encourage it to wake up. Some Japanese companies are capitalizing on this knowledge by pumping specific essential oils such as lemon through the air-circulating systems of their offices, in order to increase productivity in their workers. Essential oils can also help balance mental or emotional states. Get to know some of the oils in the list below, and use them to create emotional balance in your environment.

Emotional ecology

- **Basil** Banishes fear and indecision and clarifies the mind.
- **Cedarwood** Cleanses the mind and heightens creativity.
- **Chamomile** Calms panic and hysteria, good for insomnia.
- **Clary Sage** Clears head after mental activity.

- **Geranium** Relieves anxiety and depression.
- **Jasmine** Helps counter shyness.
- **Lavender** Calms irritability and impatience.
- **Lily** Restores energy.
- **Neroli** An anti-shock aid, heightens mental functions.
- **Peppermint** Uplifts the spirits, counters apathy.
- **Rosemary** A good nerve tonic.
- **Sandalwood** Helps open the mind to new ways of thinking.
Ylang Ylang An anti-depressant and aphrodisiac.

Aromatics in practice

- Use an essential oil burner or diffuser to fill your room with energy-enhancing scent molecules. We particularly like the electrical Aroma-Stream by Tisserand (see Resources, p.136). It fans the oils into the air without distorting them with heat. A simple diffuser comes in the form of a ring which you place around a light bulb. The heat of the bulb causes the oils to evaporate into the atmosphere. (But, like any heat-diffuser, it does destroy some of the power of the essence.)
- You can make your own diffuser by putting 8-10 drops of essential oils on a small piece of cardboard or in a dish of warm water and leaving it on a warm radiator or Aga stove.
- Carry aromatics with you by scenting a handkerchief with a few drops of oil. You can inhale the beneficial properties whenever you feel the need, for instance when you are in a stuffy or smoky room.
- Keep a collection of a few basic oils such as rosemary, lavender, sandalwood, geranium and neroli

in your bathroom and let them remind you to take long, soothing aromatic baths. Remember to add the oils just before you get in (so that they don't evaporate too quickly). For a normal-size bath use 10-15 drops. Remember that several oils combined can create a positive synergistic effect.

Water wonders

An essential oil-bath can provide you with another bonus – the restorative properties of the water itself. No matter how excited we are by some of the latest high-tech treatments for enhancing energy, we remain loyal devotees of hydrotherapeutic practices.

Hydrotherapy, made famous by the German physician Kneipp in the nineteenth century, makes use of the electrical properties of water to improve the electromagnetic balance in your body. Most hydrotherapy practices involve the application of alternating hot and cold water. This increases the electrical charge or the 'aliveness' of each of the body's cells which in turn stimulates the body's systems into activity (such as the lymphatic system responsible for clearing wastes).

A simple way to incorporate hydrotherapy into your daily routine is to finish a warm bath or shower with a 30-45 second cold shower. Doing this first thing in the morning can set your system into action for the day ahead or revive you after a relaxing evening bath and get you ready for a night out. For extra help, alternate between the warm and cold 2 or 3 times – a minute or two of warm to 30 seconds of cold – finishing with the

cold. It's important that you wrap up well afterwards, particularly if you are sensitive to the cold. Daily hydrotherapy can help improve circulation and make you more resistant to cold temperatures, but you need to go gently at the beginning.

The dew bath
Another hydrotherapy trick which we adore is barefoot walking on dewy grass. Thanks to the reflexology points on the soles of the feet, such a treatment can stimulate all the organs in your body. It is especially good for improving intestinal function and relieving congestion in the head and chest. Start by rubbing your feet with a wet cloth for a minute or two, then put on socks and shoes and walk about. After a few times, try walking barefoot on dry grass and then wet. If you don't have a garden, take the treatment when you can – either in a park or out in the country. Barefoot walking is also a good way to connect with the rich energy of the earth beneath you.

Soothing sounds

The final external element for creating a core-nurturing cocoon is sound. Just as aromatic essences can alter your emotional state, so too can sound. The sound of running water, for instance, winding its way over stones in a stream, has a remarkable ability to cleanse the mind of worries, leaving you feeling calm and clear. The sound of a heart beat played in an infant's cot can reassure her and send her into blissful sleep. You can take advantage of the sounds of nature in the form of cassettes which reproduce the breaking of waves or the calling of birds. Certain new age musical tapes can also be profoundly soothing, although others are aggravating. Take a Walkman to a shop which sells them and insist on trying them out before you buy. We like to work in a room with 'live' sound in the form of wind chimes. They create a soothing background environment that can help counter stress. It is important to find chimes that harmonize with one another. The most soothing sounds, according to expert Steven Halpern, are produced by aluminium or copper tubular chimes measuring 12" – 18" in length.

Internal enhancers

Dynamic women who drive themselves to achieve superhuman feats and continually endure high stress levels eventually burn out and get sick. They ignore one of the most important principles in creating endless energy – the gentle energy of restoration. There is something very inviting about a fast-paced, buzzy lifestyle that keeps your adrenalin pumping and your mind racing. Like many women, we sometimes find ourselves caught up in the excitement of such a pace, only realizing we have overdone it when we become completely exhausted. Because of this tendency, we try to make a practice of finding 'soft time' each day to restore ourselves. This can be 10-30 minutes of mediation, a 30-minute afternoon nap or even guided imagery using a relaxation tape. There are also

certain days when, for whatever reason, the body just doesn't feel like being pushed. This may be due to the phase of the moon, or the weather or our own biological cycles. It is important to be sensitive to such rhythms and treat yourself with gentleness accordingly if you possibly can. When you do, you discover that these 'soft days' can be full of richness and creativity which goes unnoticed if you are charging around being 'efficient'.

Slumbering secrets

The body has its own built-in restoring mechanism – sleep. People that boast how few hours sleep they can get away with forget that many essential processes take place during sleep. One of the great minds of our time – Einstein – could sleep for 12 or more hours at a stretch. It is at rest that your body repairs and rebuilds its cells and eliminates cell wastes. Sleep also helps clear out mental or emotional wastes through the process of dreaming.

Blissful sleep

A good night's sleep as Shakespeare knew can 'knit up the ravell'd sleeve of care'. The problem is that sleep is not something you can *try* to get. As any insomniac knows, no amount of wishing and wanting can guarantee peaceful repose. Sleeping involves a mode which many dynamic women know little about – that of *allowing* rather than 'doing'. This sense of *letting it happen* is a key to drawing upon life's softer energies. Learning to let go, soften and allow is what

resourcing energy from within is all about. Here are some helpful ways to encourage the allowing mode of sleep.

Insomnia socks

One of the most unusual and effective hydrotherapy remedies for the restless is the wet socks trick. Next time counting sheep fails, try this instead. Take a pair of short cotton socks and soak them in cold water. Wring them out well and put them on your feet. Then cover your feet with a second pair of dry socks – either wool or cotton – and retire for the night. The cool socks on your feet will help to draw the energy in your body downwards, leaving you feeling calm and relaxed.

Herbal help

Several herbs act as safe and natural tranquillizers which can help relax your mind and body for sleep. One of the most popular is passion flower or passiflora which can be bought in tablet form. Others include hops, valerian root and skullcap. You can swallow them in pill/capsule form or make a herbal tea nightcap. The classic one is chamomile. Another tasty nightcap is a tablespoon of orange flower water stirred into a cup of hot water with a little honey.

Bedtime snacks

Although it is best not to go to bed on a full stomach, some people find it helpful to have a little something before retiring. Some foods help promote sleep because they contain high quantities of the amino acid tryptophan – a precursor to the calming brain chemical serotonin –

or because they encourage the conversion of tryptophan to serotonin. Other foods taken at bedtime can disrupt sleep because they contain high quantities of tyramine which increases the release of noradrenaline – a brain chemical that excites the nervous system.

Good sleep foods

Bananas, figs, dates, yogurt, tuna, whole grain crackers, nut butter, turkey.

Bad sleep foods

Caffeine, alcohol, sugar, cheese, chocolate, sauerkraut, bacon, ham, sausage, aubergine, potatoes, spinach and tomatoes.

Sedative scents

Try this sleepy aromatic blend in a bedtime bath: 6 drops of lavender oil, 4 drops of chamomile and 2 of neroli (orange blossom). Or put a drop or two of each of the oils on your pillow before sleep.

Write your troubles away

If you suffer from a racing mind last thing at night, it might be an ideal time to make a practice of writing in your *Endless Energy* journal. Clearing thoughts and worries out of your mind and onto the page can free you of anxiety for the night and help you surrender to a deep and satisfying sleep.

Magnet magic

If you are frequently plagued by insomnia and nothing seems to help, try a magnetic bed or pillow.

We have found both extremely helpful for ensuring deep and restorative sleep. A magnetic bed can also counter the sleep-disrupting effects of geopathic stress (caused by underground electrical and water lines). An obvious but often useful way to help overcome the problem of geopathic stress is to change the position of your bed in the room or the direction in which you sleep on your bed. Both can make a world of difference.

Core connections

A daily meditation practice gives access to energy resources from your core. Regular meditation helps improve concentration and focus so that you are able to pour all of yourself into whatever activity you undertake. It can also bring you a better sense of your own centre, providing you with a safe place to return to whenever you feel out of balance. This centre is also the source of your personal power. Anyone who experiences erratic energy ups and downs and mood swings can benefit considerably from meditating for 15-30 minutes a day.

We like to meditate sitting cross-legged on a cushion on the floor. (Raising your bottom a few inches off the ground helps align the spine and is more comfortable.) To encourage the flow of energy in the body we have adopted the Buddhist practice of placing the back of the left hand in the palm of the right one. We also find it helpful to meditate in the same place each time. Leslie has a meditation altar in the corner of her room. On it she keeps several treasured possessions as well as candles and incense.

Zen breath meditation

This is one of the simplest yet most effective forms of mediation we have found. Try to meditate for 10-15 minutes to begin with. Keep a watch or clock close by to check on the time.

Sit comfortably and close your eyes. Become aware of your breathing but don't alter it. Watch the breath come in and then out and count 'one' silently to yourself. The next time you breathe out count 'two' and so on up to ten. Then begin again at one. Keep a sense of allowing throughout the meditation so that you don't try to change your breathing pattern or anticipate the next number to come. Simply watch the ebb and flow of your breath.

Although it is simple, this meditation, as you will discover, is not easy. It is quite normal for your mind to wander off or for you to lose count. When this happens do not get upset or frustrated. Simply notice that it has happened, smile to yourself and gently bring your focus back to your breathing, beginning again at 'one'. How far you manage to count before you get distracted is completely unimportant. The numbers are simply a way to help focus your entire being on the breath.

Imaginary holiday

Whenever we feel in need of a holiday but because of commitments can't take a break, we have found it helpful to turn inwards and replenish from the resources of the inner world through the imagination. The following guided imagery journey can be made into a relaxation tape to encourage the *allowing* mode and help restore your energy levels when you become depleted. As you will remember from Chapter 3, Free Your Spirit, the use of the imagination brings about physiological changes in the body so that you can *actually* restore your body through your mind's eye.

It is best to do the guided journey lying on your back on the floor with a carpet or blanket beneath you. Place a cushion or a book under your neck and head so that your chin is parallel to the floor and your neck feels free. If you experience tightness in your lower back with your legs straight, do the exercise with your legs bent, placing your feet near your buttocks, about hip-width apart. Before you lie down, do a few gentle stretches to release any tension in your arms, shoulders, back and legs.

Use the following script to make your own guided imagery tape. Read the text in a slow relaxed way, leaving pauses wherever there are ellipses so that your mind has time to explore each image. You may need a couple of attempts at the recording to get the formula right for you.

Let's begin the journey inward. Make yourself comfortable lying on your back… Take a deep breath in and sigh out fully… Bring your awareness to the contact between your body and the floor. Allow the floor to support you fully so that your muscles can give up any sense of effort and you can simply enjoy feeling safe, supported and calm.

Become aware of your breathing. Notice how the air feels as it enters through your nostrils and travels down into your body. Notice the feeling of the air as it leaves your body again. As you inhale imagine that you breathe in peace and relaxation and as you exhale imagine breathing out any tension or worries…

Now imagine that as you inhale the breath travels all the way down to your feet, filling them like balloons. As you exhale the balloons deflate again leaving your feet completely relaxed and soft. Feel this gentle expansion and deflation in your feet with each breath… Now move your awareness to your calves. Again imagine them as balloons. As you breathe in they fill with air and as you breathe out they deflate, becoming loose and limp… Enjoy the feeling of calm at the end of an exhalation… Now breathe into your knees. Imagine them as small balloons which fill and deflate with the breath… Move up to your thighs and allow them to be filled with breath. As you breathe out, let go of any tension so that the thigh muscles become soft and loose… Imagine your pelvis as a balloon. As you breathe in feel the balloon expanding all the way around you. As you breathe out, let the balloon collapse into the floor beneath you. Feel the ease with which the balloon is filled and deflated… Now bring your awareness to the balloon of your belly and chest. Feel your ribs expanding as the balloon inflates, and as you exhale let the rib cage melt into the floor… Now bring your awareness to your hands and let your breath fill them with air. As you exhale feel your hands become soft and loose… Let your breath fill the balloons of your lower arms and elbows, leaving your arms limp and heavy on the out breath… Feel the breath in your upper arms and shoulders, loosening any tension as it flows in and leaving your arms and shoulders limp and free as it flows out… Now allow your breath to flow gently in and out of your neck and head, bringing a sense of deep relaxation and calm… Enjoy the sensation of your breath flowing throughout your entire body bringing a feeling of peace and contentment to every cell…

Now let's begin the journey inward. Become aware of your eyes and imagine them as 2 pebbles dropping backwards towards your inner world. As you follow this movement you find yourself in a tunnel with a point of light ahead of you. You move towards the light and gradually emerge into your inner garden…

The landscape is very pleasing to you. It may resemble a place you have already visited or it may be completely new to you. But this garden is part of your own inner world and you feel perfectly at home. Take a moment to admire the surroundings…

Winding through the garden is a pathway of soft, warm earth. You remove your shoes and begin to walk barefoot along the path, feeling your feet gently massaged beneath you… The sun is shining and you feel its warmth on your skin… A gentle breeze caresses your face… As you walk along the path you notice that the green of the plants in your garden is particularly intense. Just by looking at the colour you seem to absorb their life energy…

You walk through the garden and come to a place that is particularly beautiful. The flowers and trees planted here have been chosen not only for their beauty but for their fragrances. Notice your favourite flowers… Notice which colours are most pleasing… Allow the exquisite bouquet of scents to fill your lungs…

Soon you hear the sound of running water. As you follow it you come to a small river flowing into a rock pool. It is warm and you decide to bathe in the water. You undress, leaving your clothes on the mossy bank and step into the pool. The water is invigorating and as it flows over your skin your entire body feels fresh and alive…

Flowing into the pool is a stream of pure, clear water that sparkles in the sunlight. You cup your hands under the stream and drink a few sips. As the water moves down inside you it fills your body with light, cleansing you from the inside.

When you are ready, you emerge from the pool onto the bank and notice that some fresh clothes have been laid out ready for you. Notice what colour and style they are… As you put them on how does the material feel against your skin? Now look around you for the most comfortable place to sit and relax. Remember this is your garden and you can create anything you like to suit your needs… Move to your perfect spot and sit or lie down… Imagine that you close your eyes and drop down to the source of life within you. Allow any thoughts or images to arise spontaneously from this place inside and just enjoy watching them as they do…

(Leave a few minutes' silence.)

When you are ready to leave your inner world and come back to the room in which you are lying, simply imagine yourself back in the tunnel of your mind. Let your awareness drift slowly upwards towards your eyelids. Take a couple of deep breaths… Stretch gently and open your eyes.

Chapter 12

Myths *for* power

In the universe, in your own life, only one thing is constant: *change*. Change is the very essence of life itself. The tides change, the moon changes, the seasons change in cyclic patterns. Day becomes night and night day again. A seed opens, grows, becomes a plant, then flowers and produces fruit. Like you, to unfold in all its magnificence, it must first survive. And the only way a living thing can defy that famous law of *entropy* and survive is by changing.

There are two kinds of change: simple change where, whatever has changed can always change back again, and *transformation*, where the change that takes place is one-way and there is no going back. It is through transformation that a seed (or a woman) at a lower level of life order is changed into the same seed or woman at a higher one. By making such transformative changes in our lives the potential embodied in our own seedpower is set free to unfold in all its splendour. And it is in learning to work *with* the transformative energies in our lives that we release endless energy. We allow change to empower us.

Working with transformation is seldom easy. The one-way nature of transformational change demands that you pass through a period of confusion where old structures disintegrate in order to make reorganization at a higher order possible. Such change can be very unsettling. This is true not only in human terms but throughout the universe.

Nobel Prize winner Ilya Prigogine has shown that for any system in the universe to evolve from one level of order to a higher level it has to pass through a period of chaos. Evidence of this kind of transformational change can be seen all around us – in the metamorphosis of a caterpillar to a butterfly and in the growth of a fertilized egg into a baby. We hear of it in our myths. It is told in the Christian story of crucifixion followed by resurrection and in the tale of the phoenix who, consumed by flames, rises out of the fire to soar again in greater splendour. We see it in our own bodies when a healing crisis takes place, and wastes we have carried for years rise to the surface creating temporary symptoms only to be lifted off to make way for healing.

The fires of change

With transformation as leitmotif of all life, you would think we would all know how to cope with it. Yet getting through periods of disorganization and the dissolving of limitations in our lives in order to grow is the most difficult task any of us ever faces. It asks that a woman commit to the flames anything which, no matter how useful in earlier times, has become outmoded. This means everything that no longer serves her – ideas, habits, old thought patterns, emotions from the past and, most important of all, any of her living patterns which have their roots in *fear*. Her metamorphosis demands that these things be laid upon an altar and sacrificed so that life can then re-create itself out of the ashes in a higher form.

The word *sacrifice* means to make sacred. It does not mean, as so often in our culture it is taken to mean, ripping oneself apart, or denying oneself. The idea of sacrificing something which has outstayed its welcome or is no longer useful sounds as though it should be easy – rather like cleaning out a cupboard. But when it is happening it can be terrifying. It can feel as though it is *we* who are being sacrificed. This is why we fight so hard against change and find it so terrifying.

The key to riding the waves of transformation, which we as women are being asked to ride throughout our lives, is learning to make such sacrifices *willingly* – to go *with* the transformational energies when they come. When you can, then the process of transformation, instead of making you feel like the very flesh of your body is being stripped away, becomes an exciting voyage of discovery – a voyage which, although it has its perils and its pleasures, you know is taking you to a richer land. One thing keeps us from being able to do this, and that is fear.

Fear of wholeness

Fear is an essential emotion. It registers any situation in which the integrity of mindbody is threatened. Without it we would not survive. If an elephant stampedes towards you and you don't feel afraid you might not get out of its way and you'll be trampled to death. This kind of fear is *appropriate*. You identify yourself as the thing in the way of the elephant and the elephant as a threat to yourself and you take action to avoid disaster. The immune system which protects your body from illness and degeneration works in very much the same way. It recognizes *self* as opposed to *non-self* and makes sure that the integrity of self is not breached by anything that could cause it harm.

But fear has a negative side too. This same tendency to identify self from non-self for the protection of life gets turned inside out and becomes distorted. Then,

instead of serving the essential but limited purpose of preserving life for which fear is intended, it becomes a fear of life, a fear of change, the kind of fear which makes you hold on desperately to things and people and ideas and images of yourself which your life would be better without. This kind of fear is the biggest toxin that ever needs to be eliminated from your life if you want to live with endless energy and let your life unfold in all its richness and meaning.

When fear grows toxic

Toxic fear has many different faces: a fear of illness, of death, of losing a relationship, of injury, even of freedom – the very thing you want most. When toxic fear is present it pollutes your thoughts and feelings. It can produce depression, anxiety, hate, resentment and hopelessness. It also deadens relationships and makes life seem meaningless.

The reason we try so hard to hang on to everything is that we *identify* ourselves with these things – ideas, people, images of ourselves, money, a house, a job. If any of these things should be dissolved or threatened or lost in the process of change in which we are involved, we fear that we ourselves will be lost.

Every form of toxic fear is a fear of losing your *self*. And the irony of it all is that the self which you so greatly fear losing, is always some *outmoded* self – which in the process of transformation needs to be sacrificed to make way for a new, expanded, more creative self to take its place.

To live with endless energy, one needs to learn to go *with* the process of one's own unfolding – the process of *becoming* who you are. You need to go *beyond* fear. You need to move into the realm of trust – a trust in your core, in that greater self – the individual brand of energy from which every aspect of your life is nurtured and regenerated.

At the core of you

This self which lies at your core is unlimited, all-inclusive and infinitely capable of transformation. Like the leaf painted with one brush stroke by the Zen master, it is a unique microcosmic expression of the universe. So long as your sense of who you are is identified with the smaller self and all its mental and physical baggage, transformation remains an agony. However, when you begin to see that this day-to-day self is only a minute expression of your larger self from which your core energy comes, and you can begin to identify with that instead, then the whole game changes. Instead of being plagued by fear and the other negative emotions which accompany it (emotions which play a large part in the development of disease incidentally) you start to act from trust and to experience yourself as an integral and harmonious part of the all that is.

All of this takes patience and time. It also requires a conscious effort to identify and weed out outdated thought and behaviour patterns, energetic imbalance or internal pollution in the body, and to replace reactions rooted in fear with trust. This in turn calls for an internal revolution in consciousness as well as learning skills in managing change. Many of the techniques, information, ideas and exercises in this book are designed to help with both. We hope they will prove useful to you in your own journey. Use those that do. Those that do not, discard. For your journey is different from every path that has ever been walked. Each of us has to find her own way. That is the challenge of endless energy and that is the fun of it all. That is also the hero's journey in every mythology in the world.

Myth, magic and transformation

Myths have power. A myth is far more than a story. It is a tale which resonates with meaning far beyond that which the conscious mind can grasp. It evoking feelings and awareness of the interrelatedness of the smaller self and the greater self – between the individual and life as a whole. Being aware of myths which seem especially relevant to your life at any particular time can bring a sense of meaning to events or experiences which are hard to make sense of. The myth of the hero's journey can be particularly helpful in learning the art of handling transformations. It can help us approach the experience of chaos with more security since it gives structure to what is essentially an experience of the dissolution of structures – an experience where old forms and worldviews are destroyed to make way for new ones. As such, hero myth can create the safe cocoon in which the caterpillar dissolves into white gel before being metamorphosed into a butterfly.

The myth of the hero comes in as many forms as there are cultures out of which these tales have grown. It describes beautifully the archetypal process of transformation. It gives us the opportunity of playing out our own transformations in a way that offers order and

the control of ritual in which the world of space and time and the world of eternity interpenetrate. It can help replace the experience of toxic fear in the face of change with a great space into which one's daily life can become illuminated by the eternal.

The myth of the hero, no matter where it comes from or from what period of history, goes something like this. The hero is usually someone whose life works well in the family and social context in which he or she lives yet who has a yearning for something greater. She hears a call to adventure. The call can come from outside in the form of a request from someone or something or it can arise from within as an inner imperative – a message from her core. In any cast it tells her, 'Wake up, there is something more to life than can be found in the way you are living it.' The call resonates deep into her being where it remains until it is either silenced by other voices which will not allow her the freedom of following her own heart, or until the hero acknowledges its worth and sets out on her journey.

Of course every call sets up resistance at first. For the status quo in your life – your job, your relationship, the place you live, your obligations – all have to be acknowledged before the hero can begin her journey.

She sets out. Along the road helpers appear – animals, guides and friends, who warn her of dangerous places and encourage her in her quest. At some point a spirit guide arrives bringing with it some instrument of power to arm her in her tests within the mysterious land in which she walks and to help her do battle at the gateway to the new world. Cinderella is given a ball gown by her fairy godmother; Luke Skywalker is given a light sword by Obi Ben Kenobi; Athena hands Perseus her shield to protect him.

Armed with her talisman, the hero proceeds onwards towards the threshold of adventure. This is usually a tunnel, a gateway, an opening into a dark forest which leads to another world. There she meets a dragon, a monster, a guardian of the threshold, which represents the second level of resistance – the self-sabotaging and self-destructive forces in her own consciousness – which she needs to confront and conquer. On being defeated, sometimes the monster itself becomes transformed into helpmate and accompanies her into the most mysterious of all the inner worlds.

Here at the enchanted world of the mysterium tremendium she comes upon all things new and strange. But strengthened by having done battle with her enemy, and wielding her instrument of power, she feels herself capable of dealing with anything that appears. Appear it does in the form of a supreme ordeal which she must encounter. A monumental struggle ensues in which she emerges triumphant. Only now, after this, does she earn the reward of her journey – the treasure, the Grail, the inner mystical union which she has been seeking. It is the golden dawn that comes after a dark night of struggle. She has won the gift of life which heals all wounds and banishes all fear. Then, leaving the magical world behind but carrying her gift, the hero returns. Her journey has been completed. She herself has been renewed, reborn. She is coming home with greater strength, new understanding and a sense of inner fullness with which now her ordinary life will become endowed. She has passed through the process of transformation and emerges a magnificent butterfly.

Power for transformation

Each time we hear such a journey described it echoes in the deepest realms of our being. It carries with it the resonant power of transformative energy that transcends toxic fear in our own life passages. Master of mythology, the late Joseph Campbell, described the journey of the hero as the journey of the ego or the self's search for self. That is why it has so much meaning in the process of health – of becoming who you really are – and value in the quest for endless energy.

Explore myths – see which ones hold particular power for you. They may change from one period to another in your life; as you change and grow you will seek new myths. They can be enormously empowering. There is one myth which, above all others, seems to us important for women. Because of our cultural conditioning we tend to undervalue the feminine within us – that part which is instinctual, non-moral, full of feeling and irrational will. Because the society in which we live is so frightened of these things and frightened of the unconscious mind in all its myriad facets, we ourselves fear the feminine within us (which of course exists in both men and women) and judge it harshly. We swallow our anger even when it is righteous anger, we put our needs and wants below those of others. We crush our spirits. We judge ourselves wrong and we see ourselves as ugly. In doing so we dissipate our power and dishonour our core energy.

Only when the irrational feminine is embraced and its will is honoured can any of us, men or women, complete the hero's journey and return in wholeness. The most difficult task most of us ever come up against is that of accepting the part of ourselves which we find most ugly and loathsome. The best kept secret for endless energy is this: *locked within what we most hate or fear about ourselves lies our greatest power for transformation.* But let the tale be told in myth. The story of The Loathly Lady from the Arthurian Grail myths is so much more powerful than ordinary words could ever be.

Meet the hag

One Christmastide Arthur rode out with his knights to hunt. By chance he became separated from his companions and found himself at the edge of a great brackish pond. There a knight in black armour emerged from the shadows and challenged him to a fight. Arthur reached to draw his sword Excalibur and call on its power to protect him from all harm. Alas, he had come away from court without it. He could feel every ounce of strength drain away from his body in the presence of the dark and evil stranger who raised his sword and threatened to kill him. Being a responsible king, of course, Arthur told the dark knight he didn't think that killing him was such a great idea – he had a country to rule after all and knights to look after. Where would *they* be without him? The stranger, bored at the thought of such an easy kill relented and replied, 'Okay, I won't kill you so long as you return to this place in three days with the answer to a riddle I shall give you. If you fail in this task, then I shall remove your head in one full sweep.'

Arthur agreed. He figured that given half a chance and a mug or two of fancy mead, his pals back at the castle would be sure to come up with something. The riddle the stranger posed was this: 'What does every woman want?' So Arthur headed home to ask all of his knights and wise men to give him the answer. Everyone from Merlin to a goose girl he met had a go. Each gave him a different answer: 'A woman wants beauty,' said one. 'A woman wants power,' said another, or fame, or jewels, or sanctity. None could agree.

Time was running out. Finally, although he had done his best to hide from his beloved Guinevere the seriousness of the situation, the third morning arrived. Bound by his word of honour to the Black Knight, Arthur had to face the music. Along the road to the meeting at the brackish waters Arthur came upon an old woman. She sat on a tree stump by the side of the road calling his name.

Arthur dismounted and approached her with all the courtesy he could muster. For the closer he came the more ghastly this old hag appeared. Although she was dressed in fine silk and wore magnificent jewels on her gnarled and twisted hands, she was unquestionably the most hideous thing he had ever seen – or dreamed of for that matter. Her nose was like a pig's, her mouth was huge, toothless and dribbling. What hair remained on her head was greasy, and the skin all over her misshapen body was covered in oozing sores.

Arthur swallowed hard, forcing himself not to have to look away. 'My Lord,' she said in a surprisingly gentle voice, 'Why look you so dismayed?' Summoning up all his chivalrous training, Arthur apologized for his manner, trying to explain it away by telling her he was most unsettled at the prospect of returning to meet his death at the hand of an evil knight because he could not tell him the answer to the riddle, 'What does every woman want?'

'Ah,' said the hag. 'I can tell you that. But such knowledge cannot be given without payment.' Arthur, hoping once again for a reprieve from death, replied, 'Of course, Madam, anything you desire shall be yours for the answer – even half my kingdom.'

The Loathly Lady made Arthur bend down while she whispered a few words in his ear. The moment Arthur heard them, he knew his life and his kingdom had been saved. He was about to leap on his horse again and ride off to meet the stranger when she tugged on his cloak and said, 'Now I want my reward.' 'Of course, Madam, what is it that you want?' he asked. 'I want to be the wife of your bravest knight and live at your court.' Arthur, who only a moment before had felt his spirits soar, was plunged into the deepest despair. How could he possibly expect any knight to consent to marry such a hideous hag? And what would it be like to have to endure such ugliness every day at court?

'But Madam, that is impossible!' he said. The words slipped through his lips before he could catch them. Aghast at his own lack of courtesy and agonized by having to ask any of his knights, Arthur said, 'I beg your pardon, Madam. You are quite right. Come to court tomorrow. There waiting for you will be your future husband.' So saying, he mounted his horse and rode off to meet the Black Knight to convey to him the answer to the riddle.

When he got back to the castle, Arthur was distraught. The knights questioned him. He confessed that he had won his life from the Black Knight but then told them at what cost and reported his promise to the Loathly Lady. 'My very honour is at stake,' said Arthur, wringing his hands, 'unless one of you will agree to wed her.' His knights were horrified at the prospect and tried to avoid his gaze. But one – the youngest knight of all – Sir Gawain, the most courageous and purest of heart stood up. 'Worry, not my liege,' Gawain said, 'I shall save you, I will marry the woman no matter what her mien.'

Gawain did not have long to wait before he rued his offer. The marriage was planned for the following morning and the hag arrived at court. When he looked upon her, even Gawain with all his chivalry, did not know how he could go through with the ceremony. It demanded every ounce of his courage. Somehow he managed it. But things got worse. When the festivities were over, the couple were obliged to retire to their chamber for the night. Gawain, unable to face the hideousness of his wife, sat for long hours in their bedchamber with his back to the lady, writing at his desk and praying she would go to sleep without him. Was he to spend the rest of his life shackled to such a hideous monster?

Long past midnight, as the candle burnt low, he felt a hand come to rest upon his shoulder. 'Will you not come to bed now, my Lord?' a voice whispered from behind him. Shuddering with horror, Gawain mustered his courage to look at her. To his astonishment there stood not the ugly hag he had married but the most beautiful woman he had ever seen. She had golden hair and ivory skin. 'Why do you seem so surprised, My Lord?' she said to him. 'I am indeed your wife. I was enchanted by a wicked magician. But now the enchantment is half broken by your having consented to marry me and so I stand before you now in my true form.' Gawain could not believe his luck.

'Half broken?' he asked. 'Yes, my lord' was the reply. 'Sadly I am only allowed to spend half the time in my true form. For the rest I must return to the shape of the same hag which this afternoon you married. And now you must choose, my Lord. Would you have me be my true self at night when we are alone together and the hag during daylight hours?' Gawain, whose mind was flooded with passion at the thought of her beauty filling his bed each night, replied eagerly, 'Yes, that is certainly how it must be.'

In the eye of his beautiful lady appeared a tear. 'But Sir,' she said, 'Would you then have me suffer the humiliation of the court who cannot conceal their horror at my ugliness?' Now Gawain, if he was nothing else, was compassionate. He could not bear to bring this beautiful woman a tear of sorrow. 'No, of course not,' he replied. 'It shall be the other way round, of course. You shall be my beautiful wife for the court during daylight hours and the hag at night.' But this only made the lady weep the more. 'Oh sir, would you then deny me forever the joy and pleasure of your embrace?' she asked.

Poor Gawain, who after all was but a man (and man has never found it easy to deal with woman's grief), did not know what to do. After much thought he replied, 'My lady, whatever choice I make will be the wrong one. It is therefore for *you* to choose which you prefer.'

At the sound of his words the lady threw herself into his arms in glorious laughter. 'In so saying, my Lord, you have given the right answer. You have bestowed upon me what every woman wants – *her own way*. The spell at last is broken. You will never have to look upon the hideous hag again. I am my true self and it belongs to you forever.'

Such is the power of accepting that which to ourselves is most loathsome. And such is the power of myth in reminding us of it.

Chapter 12
Workbook

Workbook *for* Myths *for* power

Now let's go back to the original questions. *Who are you? What do you want? What do you think is stopping you?* Find a clean page in your journal. Without looking at your previous answers, go through the questions again, as if you were answering each for the first time. Allow yourself full freedom in writing your answers. For instance, when considering the question *What do I want?* remember that the question is not 'what do I think is *possible*?' but 'what do I really *want*?' Give yourself as much time and space as you need in order to answer each fully.

Shifting dreams

When you finish, compare your answers with those you wrote at the beginning. Are they the same? Has your idea of yourself altered or grown? Have your desires expanded or changed?

Having a handle on where you are and where you want to go empowers your own process of unfolding. Women frequently don't stop to ask such questions. Many of us spend our lives *passively* responding to the needs of others or to external demands rather than *actively* choosing to create the life we want. A few even find it hard to imagine that they are *allowed* to want anything.

At first it can be difficult to hear the small inner voice of your own being or even to believe there is a voice waiting to be heard. This comes step by step when you honour your inner imperatives as they *do* begin to present themselves. And it doesn't matter a bit whether these happen to be desires for simple things, like a wish for a pair of red shoes and the desire to learn to sing, or vast dreams of working with children in the Third World and visions of political activism.

Structural engineering

The questions can be useful in other ways too. Working with them teaches the art of creating something out of nothing. Your answers can help you learn structural engineering – the art of building bridges strong enough to carry your visions, hopes and dreams out of your inner world across the gap of uncertainty into everyday reality. But for this part you need to go back to your journal and answer one more question:

Where am I right now in relation to what I want?

To create what you want in your life – from greater self-esteem to your dream home – you need two things: to have as clear a vision as possible of what it is you are seeking and to be aware of where you are right now in relation to that vision. Being able to see both at the same time sets up a creative tension which draws you, via all the necessary intermediary steps, inexorably towards your goals. The greater your desire to achieve a goal and the clearer you can be about where you are in relation to that goal, the easier the art of creation becomes.

Knowing where you are right now is crucial. Every journey begins with just one step. Only when you stand on firm ground, having accepted reality – whether pleasant or unpleasant – can you skilfully plot a course to take that first step. This is true whether your vision be of red shoes, a new body or a new world. Living this way day by day, aware of both your current reality and your dreams, creates an incredible vortex of creative energy on which you can draw, as well as the space out of which your dream can be born.

Start small

Some wants are grandiose, others quite humble. Start with a desire you believe is within your reach and set yourself the goal of achieving it. When you have it, choose another and do the same again. Doing this over and over opens up the channels between your inner and outer worlds and brings in its wake a powerful trust in the art of creation. Gradually you come to trust your own power to make the life you want.

Beginning small can lead to great things without your feeling overwhelmed in the process. This idea is expressed beautifully in a short story by the American writer Carson McCullers:

I meditated on love and reasoned it out. I realized what is wrong with us. Men fall in love for the first time. And what do they fall in love with?… A woman… Without science, with nothing to go by, they undertake the most dangerous and sacred experience in God's earth. They fall in love with a woman… They start at the wrong end of love… Can you wonder it is so miserable?…Do you know how love should begin? A tree. A rock. A cloud.

(Collected Stories, Houghton Mifflin Company, Boston, 1987)

Woundings transmuted

And what about the distortions in seedpower which each of us has to deal with? The most powerful of all our distortions are locked within a woman's deepest woundings. Here are to be found her greatest weaknesses but also her greatest strengths.

Your woundings are like crystals entwined in the roots of a growing plant. Crystals work in two ways: either they absorb water and life-enhancing nutrients from the plant, starving it of sustenance, or they dissolve to feed the plant with their richness and increase its strength.

Our deepest woundings, fed on the energy of negative beliefs, cripple us. Gradually allowed to become conscious, honoured and then forgiven, they bring about our greatest healing. Woundings can also help you to set your course ahead. Like the experience of crisis, given patience and acceptance, woundings are transmuted into power. Work with them. Continue to write in your journal and to listen silently to the inner promptings of your heart while you are still in meditation or walking beneath green trees. It is in the silence of nothingness that the seeds of all our creations are sown.

When in doubt remember the Axolotl:

Axolotls are dull, stupid animals. They look like enormous tadpoles, six inches long. People used to keep them in tanks in their sitting rooms. There the axolotls blundered about, not looking, not caring, not even wondering.

Yet because they grew up, had children, and grew old, people said, 'Well, that's how axolotls are and always will be.'

Salamanders are quite different. They are lively lizards, who love sun and light. They see clearly where they are going, and run wherever they please, relishing life.

One day a scientist discovered that if an axolotl is given the right food and right kind of help, it changes and turns into what it was always meant to be – a SALAMANDER!

(From Leila Berg's Introduction to Being Me and Also Us by Alison Stallibrass, Scottish Academic Press, Edinburgh, 1989)

Resources

Bach flower remedies: from homeo-pathic chemists and health food stores.

Calcium and magnesium: Calcium EAP-2 and Magnesium EAP-2 by Biocare, available by post from BioCare, 17 Pershore Road South, Birmingham B30 3EE. Tel 021 433 3727, Fax 021 433 3879. Nature's Own also do an excellent calcium and magnesium available from health food stores.

Digestive enzymes: Digest Aid by BioCare (see above).

Epsom salts: order household grade in 7lb bags from a chemist.

Essential oil diffuser: The Aroma-Stream available by post from Tisserand Aromatherapy Products Ltd, Knoll Business Centre, Old Shoreham Road, Hove, Sussex BN3 7GS. Tel 0273 412 139

Evening primrose oil: Nature's Own do a very good pure Evening Primrose Oil (not a blend) which is cold pressed, free from herbicides or pesticides, and non-solvent extracted. It is sold in capsules, and also in a liquid dropper for vegetarians from Nature's Own, 203-205 West Malvern Road, West Malvern, Worcs WR14 4BB. Tel 0684 892 555, Fax 0684 892 643

Flaxseed oil or linseed oil: use only cold pressed in a bottle or in capsule available by post from Nature's Own (see above). Must be kept in refrigerator at all times and used within a few weeks (see sell-by date on package).

Free form amino acids: L-glutamine, L-tyrosine etc by Solgar from good health food stores.

Full-spectrum lighting: office lighting systems available from Spectra Lighting, York House, Lower Harlestone, Northampton NN7 4EW, Tel 0604 821 904, Fax 0604 821 902. Sun boxes, bulbs, tubes, etc available from Wholistic Research Company (see below). Light boxes available from Environmental Office Systems, 6 Victoria House, 121 Longacre, London WC2E NPA

Glycophos energy supplement: available by post from Health Innova-tions, Unit 10, Riverside Business Centre, Brighton Road, Shoreham, West Sussex BN43 6RE. Tel 0273 440 177, Fax 0273 465 325

Hand massage tools and anti-cellulite cosmetics: Elancyl do a good all-in-one treatment called MP24, complete with creams. Shiseido have an excellent lotion product in their Essential Energy range which comes in a special nobbly bottle that you use as a massage glove. Clarins do their own massage device which you can use together with their Multi-Actif Body Shaping Lotion. Cellutherapie by Clairol is an electrical vibromassage system complete with massage oil and smoothing lotion.

Herbs: Solgar do a fine range of encapsulated herbs such as comfrey, echinacea, valerian, fo-ti, suma, etc which are clean and have been carefully processed and packaged to preserve their wholeness (they also do an excellent Co-Enzyme Q10). Good herbs are available by post from Gerard, 3 Wickham Road, Bournemouth, Dorset BH7 6JX. Tel 0202 434 116, Fax 0202 417 079. (Stay away from any herbal products which have been irradiated, and be careful about buying herbs in bulk – too many these days are replete with pesticides and herbicides.)

Herb teas: some of our favourite blends include Cinnamon Rose, Orange Zinger and Emperor's Choice by Celestial Seasonings; Warm and Spicy by Symingtons; Blackcurrant Bracer or Golden Slumbers by The London Herb and Spice Co; Creamy Carob French Vanilla Yogi tea by Golden Temple Products is a strong spicy blend, perfect as a coffee replacement.

Ionizers: many good models for desk, home, car, etc. are available by post from Wholistic Research Company, Bright Haven, Robin's Lane, Lolworth, Cambridge CB3 8HH. Tel 0954 781 074

Magnetic beds and magnets: the best-quality beds, pillows and magnets for personal use by post from Biomagnetics UK, 315 Chorley New Road, Bolton BL1 5BP. Tel 0204 497 239

Marigold swiss vegetable bouillon: this instant broth powder based on vegetables and sea salt is available from health food stores or direct from Marigold Foods, Unit 10, St Pancreas Commercial Centre, 63 Pratt Street, London NW1 0BY. Tel 071 267 7368. It comes in regular and low-salt forms. The low-salt form is excellent for making spirulina broth.

Multivitamin and mineral supplements: Multivitamin & Multimineral Tablet made by Nature's Own or VM 2000 from Solgar – both available from good health food stores. Tel Nature's Own 0684 892 555 or Solgar 0494 791 691 for stockists nearest you.

Natural fibre blend: Colenz includes psyllium seed, psyllium husks, pectin, flaxseed and lactobacillus acidophilus, alginates, etc. from good health food stores or by post from Health Innovations (as above).

Powdered psyllium husks: available from good health food stores or by post from Green Farm, Burwash Common, East Sussex TN19 7LX. Tel 0435 882 482

Propolis: Comvita have a range of propolis products including capsules, tincture, lozenges, toothpaste, ointment, elixir and mouthwash, available from The New Zealand Natural Food Company Ltd, 9 Holt Close, Highgate Wood, London N10 3HW. Tel 081 444 5660

Rebounder units: the best quality rebounders come from PT Leisure Ltd, New Rock House, Dymock, Gloucestershire GL18 2BB. Tel 0531 890 888. (Cheaper versions often wear out quickly or break.) A ring-bound book called 'Rebound Training' which includes exercise routines for beginners through to advanced enthusiasts is also available from PT Leisure.

Sea plant complex: Pro-Algen available from good health food stores or by post from Health Innovations (see above).

Sea plants for cooking and salads: can be bought from Japanese grocers or macrobiotic health shops.

Silica: Kervran's Silica from good health-food stores or by post from Health Innovations Ltd (as above). Tel 0273 440 177

Single vitamins and minerals: Nature's Own do unique vitamins which through a patented process have been bonded to food proteins to render them highly bio-available and assimilable; their minerals are put through a biotec process that organically ties them to a food matrix. So special is this process of renaturing and so thorough are the studies – published and unpublished on their products – that many of their supplements are treated as unique supplements prescribable by doctors: They do an excellent Vitamin B Complex, good niacin, Beta Carotene, Niacin, Calcium, Magnesium, as well as other single vitamins and minerals, including a good chromium. For stockists nearest you, tel 0684 892 555

Skin brush: from good chemists – must have bristles of vegetable origin (not nylon)

Skin care anti-wrinkle tablets: Imedeen based on fish cartilage is available from leading chemists and health-food stores as well as direct by post from Health Innovations Ltd (as above).

Spirulina: Lifestream brand is absolutely pure from good health food stores or ordered by post from Lifestream Research Ltd, Ash House, Stedham, Midhurst, West Sussex GU29 0PT. Tel 0730 813642, Fax 0730 815 109

Tea tree oil: from health-food stores and herbalists.

Further reading

Chapter 1

Dossey, Larry, MD. *Beyond Illness: Discovering the Experience of Health*, New Science Library, Shambala, Boulder & London, 1984

Harding, M. Esther. *The Way of All Women*, Longmans Green and Co., London, 1933

Harding, M. Esther. *Woman's Mysteries: Ancient and Modern*, Rider & Co., London, 1971

Progoff, Ira. *The Practice of Process Meditation*, Dialogue House Library, New York, 1980

Chapter 2

Bateson, Gregory. *Mind and Nature: A Necessary Unity*, Flamingo, Fontana Paperbacks, Great Britain, 1980

Dossey, Larry, MD. *Space, Time and Medicine*, Shambala, Boulder & London, Colorado, 1982

Odent, Michel. *Water and Sexuality*, Arkana, Penguin Books, 1990

Parabola: Myth and the Quest for Meaning, 'Inner Alchemy', Vol.III, No.3, August 1978 and 'The Body', Vol.X, No.3, August 1985, Tamarack Press, New York

Walker, Barbara G. *The Crone: Woman of Age, Wisdom and Power*, HarperCollins, New York, 1988

Woodman, Marion. *The Owl Was a Baker's Daughter: Obesity, Anorexia Nervosa and the Repressed Feminine*, Inner City Books, Canada, 1980

Woodman, Marion. *The Pregnant Virgin: A Process of Psychological Transformation*, Inner City Books, Canada, 1985

Chapter 3

Bohm, David. *Wholeness and the Implicate Order*, Routledge & Kegan Paul, London, 1980

Bohm, David & Mark Edwards. *Changing Consciousness: A Dialogue of Words & Images*, Harper, San Francisco, 1992

Devreux, Paul, John Steele and David Kubrin. *EarthMind: Communicating with the Living World of Gaia*, Destiny Books, Rochester, Vermont, 1992

Harman, Willis, Ph.D. and Howard Rheingold. *Higher Creativity*, Institute of Noetic Sciences, Jeremy P. Tarcher, Inc., California, 1984

LeShan, Lawrence. *Holistic Health: How to Understand and Use the Revolution in Medicine*, Turnstone Press Ltd, UK, 1984

Marks, Linda. *Living With Vision*, Knowledge Systems Inc., USA, 1989

Ornstein, Robert, Ph.D. and David Sobel, M.D. *The Healing Brain: Breakthrough Discoveries About How the Brain Keeps us Healthy*, Touchstone, Simon & Schuster Inc., New York, 1987

Oyle, Irving. *Time Space and the Mind*, Celestial Arts, California, 1976

Pelletier, Kenneth R. *Towards a Science of Consciousness*, Delta, New York, 1978

White, John. *Frontiers of Consciousness: The Meeting Ground Between Inner and Outer Reality*, Julian Press, Crown Publishing, New York, 1985

Wilber, Ken. *The Holographic Paradigm and Other Paradoxes: Exploring the Leading Edge of Science*, Shambala, Boulder & London, 1982

Zukav, Gary. *The Dancing Wu Li Masters: An Overview of the New Physics*, Rider Books, Random House (UK), London, 1991

There are 2 books that we recommend for inspiration and encouragement in creative writing. The first, by Brenda Ueland, encourages the reader to discover her true self through the act of writing. The second, by Natalie Goldberg, gives fun practical tips for beginning writing as a daily practice:

Ueland, Brenda. *If You Want to Write: Releasing Your Creative Spirit*, Element Books, Dorset, 1991

Goldberg, Natalie. *Writing Down the Bones*, Shambala, Boston, 1986

Chapter 5

Brekhman, I.I. *Man and Biologically Active Substances: The Effect of Drugs, Diet and Pollution on Health,* Trans. J.H. Appleby, Pergamon Press, Oxford, 1980

Downing, Damien. *Day Light Robbery,* Arrow Books, London, 1988

Mansfield, Peter. *The Good Health Handbook: Help Yourself Get Better,* Grafton Books, Collins, London, 1988

Perera, Sylvia Brinton. *The Scapegoat Complex: Towards a Mythology of Shadow and Guilt,* Inner City Books, Canada, 1986

Selye, Hans, M.D. *Stress Without Distress,* Hodder and Stoughton, London, 1975

Selye, Hans, M.D. *The Stress of Life,* McGraw-Hill, New York, 1956

Smyth, Angela. *SAD Seasonal Affective Disorder: Who Gets It, What causes It, How To Cure It,* Unwin Paperbacks, London 1990

Soyka, Fred with Alan Edmonds. *The Ion Effect: How Air Electricity Rules Your Life and Health,* Bantam Books, 1978

Chapter 6

Leonard, Linda Schierse. *Witness to the Fire: Creativity and the Veil of Addiction,* Shambala, Boston, 1990

Chapter 7

Crook, William G. M.D. *The Yeast Connection: A Medical Breakthrough,* Professional Books, Jackson, Tennessee, 1983

Jensen, Dr Bernard, and Mark Anderson. *Empty Harvest: Understanding the Link Between Our Food, Our Immunity, and Our Planet,* Avery Publishing Group, Inc., New York,1990

Mackarness, Richard. *Chemical Victims,* Pan Books, London, 1980

Mansfield, Dr Peter and Dr Jean Monro. *Chemical Children: How to Protect Your Family from Harmful Pollutants,* Century, London, 1987

Philpott, William H. M.D. and Dwight K. Kalita, Ph.D. *Brain Allergies: The Psycho-Nutrient Connection,* Keats Publishing, Inc., New Canaan, Connecticut, 1980

Chapter 8

Bach, Edward. *The Twelve Healers and Other Remedies,* The C.W. Daniel Company Ltd, Walden, Essex, 1933

Calbom, Cherie and Maureen Keane. *Juicing For Life,* Avery, New York, 1992

Cousins, Norman. *Anatomy of an Illness as Perceived by the Patient: Reflections on Healing and Regeneration,* W.W. Norton & Company, New York, 1979

Hyne Jones, T.W. *Dictionary of the Bach Flower Remedies: Positive and Negative Aspects,* Ibid. 1976

Gray, Robert. *The Colon Health Handbook: New Health Through Colon Rejuvenation,* Rockridge Publishing Company, Oakland, California, 1980

Grof, Christina and M.D. Stanislav. *The Stormy Search for the Self: A Guide to Personal Growth Through Transformational Crisis,* Jeremy P. Tarcher, Inc., Los Angeles,1990

Grof, Christian and M.D. Stanislav. *Spiritual Emergency: When Personal Transformation Becomes a Crisis,* Jeremy P. Tarcher, Inc., Los Angeles, 1989

Joy, W. Brugh M.D. *Avalanche: Heretical Reflections on the Dark and the Light,* Ballantine Books, New York, 1990

Morgan, Elaine. *The Descent of Woman,* Souvenir Press, London, 1972

Perera, Sylvia Brinton. *Descent to the Goddess: A Way of Initiation for Women,* Inner City Books, Canada, 1932

Thrash, Agatha Moody, M.D and Calvin L. Thrash Jr. M.D. *Home Remedies: Hydrotherapy Massage Charcoal and other Simple Treatments,* Thrash Publications, Seale, Alabama, 1981

Vlamis, Gregory. *Flowers to the Rescue: The Healing Vision of Dr Edward Bach,* Thorsons, Wellingborough, Northamptonshire, 1986

Wolkstein, Diane and Samuel Noah Kramer. *Inana: Queen of Heaven and Earth: Her Stories and Hymns from Sumer,* Rider Books, London, 1984

Chapter 9

Andersen, Arden B. *The Anatomy of Life & Energy in Agriculture,* Acres USA, Kansas City, Missouri, 1989

Bircher-Benner, M. M.D. *The Prevention of Incurable Disease,* James Clarke & Co. Ltd. Cambridge, 1969

Fukuoka, Masanobu. *Road Back to Nature: Regaining the Paradise Lost,* Japan Publications, Inc., Tokyo, 1987

Grant, Doris and Jean Joice. *Food Combining for Health: A New Look at the Hay System,* Thorsons, Wellingborough, Northamptonshire, 1984

Henrikson, Robert. *Earth Food Spirulina,* Ronore Enterprises, Inc. Laguna Beach, California, 1989

Hills, Christopher, Ph.D., D.Sc. *The Secrets of Spirulina: Medical Discoveries of Japanese Doctors,* trans. Dr Robert Wargo, University of the Trees Press, Boulder Creek, California, 1980

Hurd, Frank J. and Rosalie Hurd. *A Good Cook… Ten Talents,* The College Press, Collegedale, Tennessee, 1968

Kalson, Carol and Stan. *Learn By Doing Holistic H.E.L.P Handbook,* International Holistic Center, Inc., Phoenix, Arizona, 1979

Kenton, Leslie and Susannah. *Raw Energy,* Arrow, London, 1984

Kirschner, H. E. M.D. *Nature's Healing Grasses,* H.C. White Publications, Riverside, California, 1960

Lappe, Frances Moore and Joseph Collins with Cary Fowler. *Food First: Beyond the Myth of Scarcity,* Ballantine Books, New York, 1977

McCarrison, Sir Robert. *Nutrition and Health,* The McCarrison Society, London, 1936

Pfeiffer, Ehrenfried M.D. *The Earth's Face: Landscape and Its Relation to the Health of the Soil*, The Lanthorn Press, East Grinstead, Sussex, 1988

Stitt, Paul A. *Why George Should Eat Broccoli*, The Dougherty Company, Milwaukee, Wisconsin, 1990

Switzer, Larry. *Spirulina: The Wholefood Revolution*, Bantam Books, New York, 1982

Wigmore, Ann. *The Sprouting Book*, Avery Publishing Group, Wayne, New Jersey, 1986

Wigmore, Ann. *The Wheatgrass Book*, Avery Publishing Group, Wayne, New Jersey, 1985

Chapter 10

Becker, Robert O. M.D. *Cross Currents* Jeremy P. Tarcher, Inc., Los Angeles, CA, 1990

Egli, Markus. *Rebound Training*, PT Leisure, Dymock, Gloucestershire, 1987

Eischens, Roger, John Greist and Tom McInvaille. *Run to Reality*, Madison Running Press, Bulfin, Milwaukee, 1977

Kostrubala, Thaddeus M.D. *The Joy of Running*, Pocket Books, Simon & Schuster, New York, 1977

Leonard, George. *The Ultimate Athlete*, Avon Books, New York, 1974

Stirk, John L. *Structural Fitness: The Essential Guide to Better Body Mechanics*, Elm Tree Books, Penguin, London, 1988

White, James R. PhD. *Jump for Joy*, Goldfield Books, San Diego, 1981

Chapter 11

Ackerman, Diane. *A Natural History of the Senses*, Vintage Books, Random, New York,1991

Becker, Robert O. M.D. and Andrew A. Marino, PhD. *Electromagnetism and Life*, State University of New York Press, Albany, 1982

Becker, Robert O. M.D. & G. Seldon. *The Body Electric: Electromagnetism & the Foundation of Life*, William Morrow & Co., New York, 1986

Dinshah, Darius. *Let There Be Light*, Dinshah Health Society, Malaga, New Jersey, 1985

Davis, A. R. & W. Rawls. *The Magnetic Effect*, Acres USA Kansas City, MO, 1975

Davis, A.R. & W. Rawls. *Magnetism and Its Effect of the Living System*, Acres, USA, Kansas City, MO, 1976

Davis, A.R. & W. Rawls. *The Magnetic Blueprint of Life*, Acres USA, Kansas City, MO, 1979

Gubbins, David & Jeremy Bloxham. 'The Secular Variation of the Earth's Magnetic Field', *Nature*, Volume 317, October 31, 1985

Jacobson, Edmund, M.D. *You Must Relax*, Souvenir Press, London, 1977

Macbeth, Jessica. *Moon over Water: The Path of Meditation*, Gateway Books, Bath, 1990

Macbeth, Jessica. *Sun Over Mountain: A Course in Creative Imagery*, Ibid. 1991

Nakagawa, Kyoichi, M.D. 'Magnetic Field Deficiency Syndrome and Magnetic Treatment', *Japanese Medical Journal*, No. 2745 December 4, 1976

Ott, John N. *Health and Light*, Pocket Books, Simon & Schuster, 1973

Philpott, W.H. *Biomagnetic Handbook*, Enviro-Tech Publisher, 17171 S.E. 29th, Choctaw, OK 73020, 1990

Worwood, Valerie Ann. *The Fragrant Pharmacy: A Home and Health Care Guide to Aromatherapy and Essential Oils*, Bantam Books, New York, 1991

Chapter 12

Campbell, Joseph. *The Inner Reaches of Outer Space: Metaphor as Myth and as Religion*, Harper & Row, New York, 1986

Campbell, Joseph. *The Hero with a Thousand Faces*, Bollingen Series XVII, Princeton University Press, New Jersey, 1949

Fox, Matthew. *Original Blessing*, Bear & Company, Santa Fe, New Mexico, 1983

Grof, Stanislav. *The Adventure of Self-Discovery*, State University of New York Press, Albany, 1988

Johnson, Robert A. *Inner Work: Using Dreams and Active Imagination for Personal Growth*, Harper & Row, San Francisco, 1986

Jung, Emma and Marie-Louise Von Franz. *The Grail Legend*, trans. Andrea Dykes, Coventure, London, 1980

Prigogine, Ilya and Isabelle Stengers. *Order Out of Chaos: Man's New Dialogue with Nature*, Heinemann, London, 1984

Progoff, Ira. *Life-Study: Experiencing Creative Lives by the 'Intensive Journal' Method*, Dialogue House Library, New York, 1983

Whitmont, Edward C. *Return of the Goddess*, Arkana, London, 1983

Index